PARTNERSHIP FOR HEALTH

Building Relationships Between Women
and Health Caregivers

PARTNERSHIP FOR HEALTH

Building Relationships Between Women and Health Caregivers

Christina S. Beck
Ohio University

with
Sandra L. Ragan
University of Oklahoma

and
Athena Dupre
Southeastern Louisiana University

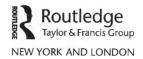 Routledge
Taylor & Francis Group

NEW YORK AND LONDON

First Published by
Lawrence Erlbaum Associates, Inc., Publishers
10 Industrial Avenue
Mahwah, New Jersey 07430

Transferred to Digital Printing 2009 by Routledge
270 Madison Ave, New York NY 10016
2 Park Square, Milton Park, Abingdon, Oxon, OX14 4RN

Library of Congress Cataloging-in-Publication Data

Beck, Christina S.
    Partnership for health : building relationships be-
tween women and health caregivers / Christina S.
Beck, with Sandra L. Ragan and Athena Dupre.
        p.   cm. — (LEA's communication series)
    Includes bibliographical references and in-
dex.
    ISBN 0-8058-2444-8 (cloth : alk. paper). — ISBN
0-8058-2445-6 (pbk. : alk. paper)
    1. Medical personnel and patient. 2. Women pa-
tients. 3. Interpersonal communication. 4. Clinical
health psychology. I. Ragan, Sandra L. II. Dupre,
Athena. III. Title. IV. Series.
R727.3.B425   1997
610.69'6—dc21   96-54801
                                            CIP

Publisher's Note
The publisher has gone to great lengths to ensure the quality
of this reprint but points out that some imperfections in the
original may be apparent.

Contents

Acknowledgments

This book marks the culmination of years of data collection and analysis as well as countless hours of engaging in conversations and reading about interpersonal communication in the women's health context. I could not begin this section without thanking Dr. Sandra L. Ragan for sparking my interest in women's health issues and in naturally occurring talk. She has inspired me, guided me, helped me, and encouraged me since we first met some 7 years ago.[1] I consider myself fortunate to have had her for my advisor during my doctorate work and incredibly lucky to have her as a very good friend and colleague.

Throughout the years in which Sandra, Athena Dupre, and I have been collecting data, we have encountered a number of women who have allowed us to audiotape conversations that occur in extremely personal contexts, such as OB-GYN examinations. We thank all of those women, both caregivers and patients, for their trust in us, their cooperation in our research, and their willingness to help others by permitting us to share their experiences. Furthermore, we thank each of the institutions in which our research took place. In an effort to protect the anonymity of our participants, we do not mention each of these institutions or participants by name here, but we extend to each of them our most sincere gratitude for making this project possible.

---

[1] "I" refers to the primary author, Christina S. Beck, when mentioned throughout the book.

We also thank our co-researchers from earlier projects. These individuals contributed to our collection of data, and although they did not participate in the writing of this book, their efforts provided us with some of the examples throughout the text. We thank Dr. Lynda Dixon Glenn Shaver for the use of the data that she collected at the Native-American health care facility as well as Dr. Michael Pagano for his assistance in gathering data at the university health care facility. We also thank Dr. Cynthia Wilkins for her work as a co-ethnographer during the ethnographic studies of two hospitals.

Although this project primarily resulted from private funding by the researchers (i.e., for the cost of audiotapes, transcription, etc.), we deeply appreciate the financial support by the Honors Tutorial College at Ohio University for the funding of a full-time summer research assistant. We are also grateful to the School of Interpersonal Communication (INCO) at Ohio University for its support of this project (i.e., the cost of photocopying, telephone conversations, postage, and secretarial support for the typing of the reference section).

Two undergraduate students at Ohio University made significant contributions to this research effort. Susan Murphy, an Honors Tutorial College student, worked tirelessly on pursuing references, chasing sources at the library, and doing preliminary transcriptions of audiotaped data. Susan truly became my "right hand" as she assisted me in obtaining information about women's health issues and in organizing that information for the proposal. I owe her an enormous debt. Betsy Hart invested a massive amount of time and energy into sorting through stack after stack of articles and books to construct the reference section. She diligently noted every citation in the text and worked to ensure that those citations appear in the reference section. The reference section exists because of her fine efforts.

Throughout the writing of this project, I have relied on the encouragement, wisdom, and expertise of my colleagues at INCO. Dr. Sue Dewine offered constant support (through her personal concern and her generosity as the director of INCO), and my other colleagues in INCO encouraged me, both personally and professionally, as I persisted in this venture. In particular, however, I thank two individuals for their willingness to read drafts of the book and to provide me with incredibly beneficial input.

Dr. Dan Modaff read drafts of the first two chapters, and he offered very valuable suggestions, usually within 24 hours! A fellow conversation analyst who is interested in the health care context, Dan helped me greatly as I fine-tuned my arguments. I thank him for his expert counsel and for his continual friendship.

I cannot adequately express my indebtedness to Dr. Roger C. Aden for his friendship and his assistance throughout the writing of this book. He volunteered to read draft after draft of the first four chapters, driving an hour from his home on one occasion just to look over my work "one more time" before I had to send the manuscript to the publisher. I thank him for his outside perspective as a rhetorician, not a health communication scholar. I thank him for the innumerable times when he gave me a synonym for a word that was being overused or a rephrasing for one of my "Garfinkel-like" sentences. I thank him for his patience as I read passages to him, prefaced only by "could ya listen to this real quick?" I thank him for his tolerance during my "tunnel vision-like preoccupation" as I completed this project. However, most of all, I thank Roger for being my best friend.

Albeit from afar, other friends and family members also supported me as I tackled this project. I thank Corinne Houghton, Michelle Boxell, Carolyn Stec, and Shari Skaggs, my friends since the eighth grade, for their ongoing friendship and our wonderful conversations about our kids, our health, our work, our memories, our dreams, and our lives. I thank my grandparents, George and Elizabeth Groscost; my mom, Sarah Beck; my sister, Teresa Kane; and my brother, Robbie Beck, for their continual support of me and my little girls.

I appreciate Jenna Riley's willingness to come to my house before and after her other job to watch my girls as I finished the last chapter, often logging 18 hour days in the process. In addition, I could not close this section without acknowledging the sacrifices that Wade Pangburn made in terms of time and professional pursuits to enable me to take the time that I needed for this project and my career. He made sure that the girls got fed, the cat litter got changed, the lawn got mowed, and the dog got walked, especially during some of my longer days.

Perhaps, most of all, however, I would like to thank my daughters, Brittany Nicole, 10, and Chelsea Meagan, 2. Although they disliked watching "Mommy" walk out of the house so often, they always greeted me with smiles upon my return. Those smiles kept me going during some of the toughest times and longest days. Even though Brittany could not understand why I would want to spend so much time writing something that was not "really interesting like a children's book," I dedicate this work to Brittany and Chelsea, my "little women," who may someday benefit from the work that has started here.

—*Christina S. Beck*

Partnership for Health:
An Introduction

Study after study suggests the existence of a grave problem in the United States that is impacting more than half of the U.S. population—the women's health care crisis. However, although the research reports are striking and shocking, statistics can easily gloss the individual trials of women patients as they strive to gain the best health care possible. Women who undergo unnecessary (but physician-recommended) hysterectomies, women who complain of classic symptoms of a heart attack but are sent home unexamined for heart problems from hospital emergency rooms, and women who do not obtain preventative screenings for cancers that are treatable if discerned early are among those who face personal trauma and tragedy because women patients have not historically been encouraged to work as partners in their own health care and because they tend to refrain from asserting themselves as partners to their health caregivers. This became more clear to me[1] when I was battling to have a second child. After 2 years of infertility, one heart-wrenching miscarriage, and agonizing and painful fertility tests, the specialist with whom I was working determined a likely source of my problem—a hormone deficiency. Because I was moving to another area, he encouraged me to tell my new obstetrician to prescribe progesterone supplements as soon as I became pregnant.

I was incredibly excited when I became pregnant soon after I moved; however, the new area was rural, and the choices for obstetricians were few. I found one doctor who would accept new patients, and in a phone conversation, I stressed that I needed to have specific tests that would follow

---

[1]"I" refers to the primary author, Christina S. Beck, when mentioned throughout the book.

my progesterone and human chorionic gonadotropin (HCG) levels. I also explained that I needed to start on the progesterone supplements immediately, as per the recommendation of my previous specialist. The doctor did agree to see me right away; however, after he examined me and looked at the papers in my file, he closed the folder and then calmly and slowly said that he would order the tests and "see how the levels come out."

I was in a panic, partly because of the emotional rollercoaster of the previous 2 years, partly because of the fear of another traumatic miscarriage, and largely because I had a great deal of trust in my former specialist and not much trust in this new doctor. An assertive woman, I sat up as straight as I could on the edge of the table, my bare legs hanging down and my chest pounding beneath the thin, pale-blue hospital gown, and I told him that I wanted and needed the progesterone supplement. I emphasized that my specialist had told me that my best chance of hanging on to a pregnancy was to begin the supplements as soon as I discovered I was pregnant. In my mind, I had already waited too long. "Honey," he said, "I'll look at the tests when they come in. Don't worry. Stress is what causes many miscarriages." He then turned, walked out the door, and left me with my mouth agape in shock and my body shaking with anger. What frustrated me the most was that I let him leave without strongly insisting that he write the prescription.

During the next 3 weeks, I returned for outpatient blood testing. With each visit, I went through the agonizing process of waiting for the lab to complete the test, waiting for the nurse to return my call with the results, waiting more tensely with each additional test to learn whether this one would show the increase that I desperately wanted to occur. I visited with the doctor on two additional occasions. On the second visit, he finally agreed that I needed a supplement and wrote the prescription. After seeing my levels only go up slightly with each test, I knew enough to know that the supplement was too late.

Eight weeks into the pregnancy, another doctor (a woman resident at the same facility) heard my frustration and ordered a sonogram to evaluate the status of the pregnancy. I was greatly moved to see the baby (whom I had already named Caitlyn) on the monitor screen and to observe her little heart pumping, fighting. The technician was not permitted to tell me anything overtly with regard to a prognosis; however, my fears were confirmed as she finally admitted that the measurements were far too small for an 8-week-old pregnancy. The technician handed me two photographs of little Caitlyn, and I stared at them as I realized that they were the only pictures that I would have of this child for my family photo album. The miscarriage started that very afternoon.

It would be easy to blame the doctor, and, to some extent, I do. However, as a normally assertive, intelligent, well-educated woman, I also take issue with the way that I responded to the interactions. I let the doctor repeatedly leave the examining room without giving me either the prescription or a satisfactory explanation of why he would not do so. I was not pleased with his treatment of my case, and yet I did not pursue a second opinion or another physician to take over my care. Implicitly, I enabled that doctor to assume the power, to take the control, to put me firmly in the rear passenger seat, and to deter me from playing the role that I wanted to play as a partner in my own care and that of my unborn child.

Hence, as I come to this issue of health care in general and of women's health care in particular, I do so with the conviction that the system often fails to produce partnerships. It fails because the individual participants do not always co-define the encounter as a collaboration nor do they always facilitate the surfacing of a multiplicity of possible relational and individual identities beyond the traditional medical model definitions of "doctor" and "patient." In my case, the doctor did not encourage a joint effort, nor did he recognize me as anyone other than someone who would just follow directives. Implicitly, he dismissed my preferred identities as an active consumer, a concerned mom, a viable participant, a partner. However, in retrospect, I realize that I did not do what was necessary to position myself as a multidimensional individual with identities and goals that encompass far more than being "just a patient" who defers, accepts, and complies.

The irony of this series of encounters is my own scholarly interest in relational communication in the women's health care context. Like William Hurt's character in the movie, *The Doctor* (a physician who develops cancer and thus becomes a patient), I found my own knowledge to be useful yet still somehow inadequate and my status as a researcher (similar to that character's status as a fellow doctor) to be treated by the doctor as insignificant and irrelevant compared to my role as patient. After this painful saga, I experienced the epiphany that participating as a partner in my own health care is much easier said than done.

The complexity of the health care encounter *and* of health care participants precludes a simplistic understanding or sound-bite-like recommendations. As communication scholars who are interested in the health care context, we must pursue that complexity. Issues like compliance gaining by doctors with their patients (see M. Burgoon et al., 1990; Davis, 1968; Hulka, Cassel, Kupper, & Burdette, 1976; Klingle & Burgoon, 1995; Korsch & Negrete, 1972; O'Hair, O'Hair, Southward, & Krayer, 1987) and communication satisfaction by patients with their health caregivers (see Buller & Buller, 1987; J. Burgoon et al., 1987; M. Burgoon, Birk, & Hall, 1991; Cardello, Ray, & Pettey, 1995; Kurata, Nogawa, Phillips, Hoffman, & Werblun, 1992; Rowland-Morin & Carroll, 1990; Stewart, 1984; Street, 1989; Street & Wiemann, 1987; Winefield & Murrell, 1991) have pervaded our interest in health care interactions (see also review by Thompson, 1990). Although research reports in those areas have provided us with rich information about those topics, they still offer only limited, narrow depictions of what occurs *between* caregivers and patients. By the nature of the research designs and questions, those studies concentrate on only one dimension, deterring a significant contribution to an understanding of the legion of social activities that transpire during the encounter or the interrelationships between those activities (see Arntson, 1985; Kreps & Query, 1990; Thompson, 1984, for calls for health communication research that explores the interactive and relational aspects of health care encounters).

Our recommendations must also embrace the implicit complexity of interaction during health care encounters instead of ignoring it. As communication scholars, we can no longer just suggest that doctors be "more responsive" or "more relationally aware" or that patients be "more assertive." In order to contribute to the ongoing dialogue about how to bring an end to the problems that women patients have historically confronted with their health care, we must pursue health care interactions in light of the multifaceted nature of those exchanges, in light of the plethora of possible relational and individual identities that caregivers and their patients may want to surface during their encounters, and in light of multiple, diverse, and potentially contradictory relational, medical, and educational goals that the interactants may have for the 10- to 15-minute visit.

To do so, we must avoid an isolated focus on *either* the caregiver *or* the patient as well as individualistic calls for a more "patient-centered" approach by caregivers or a more "consumer-oriented" approach by patients (see Hensbest & Stewart, 1990; Hunt, Jordan, Irwin, & Browner, 1989; Mishler, 1984). Experiences like mine point to the need for a better grasp of how patients and caregivers can realize a partnership dimension of their potentially multifaceted relationship. Such an understanding can only come from research that recognizes that partnerships emerge through joint, not individual, efforts. Only the dyad can communicatively co-construct a partnership orientation to the health care encounter; the responsibility does not fall on the shoulders of one or the other participant, nor does the blame. Thus, this book focuses on how women and their caregivers can interactionally co-produce a partnership dynamic, co-define their relational and individual identities, and, in so doing, co-accomplish their respective multiple goals for health care encounters.

SOCIAL CONSTRUCTION
OF HEALTH CARE ENCOUNTERS

This book stems from our concern for the health of women and from our conviction that the communication between women patients and their health caregivers is consequential to the health care experiences of women. In the following pages, we strive to attain an understanding of the complex, multifaceted nature of women's health care encounters by viewing those encounters as ongoing social constructions that may not be staticly or singularly defined. Far from "cookie-cutter-like" encounters where roles are set and pre-scripted, we contend that each health care visit is unique, emergent, and socially constructed through the communicative activities of the participants, borrowing from the social constructivist perspective advanced by Berger and Luckmann (1966) and echoed in works by Schutz (1970) and Garfinkel (1967; see also the work of Emerson, 1970, on the social construction of multiple realities in the gynecologic exam and the work of Davis, 1988a, 1988b, on the social construction of power during health care examinations).

A treatment of the health care encounter as one-dimensional and rigidly preordained by institutionalized norms, roles, and rules disregards the powerful and pivotal nature of symbolic interaction between the caregiver and patient. Such a concentrated casting of the encounter also denies the multiplicity of possibilities in terms of how the encounter will ensue (i.e., what topics will be discussed, what procedures will be done, how decisions will be made, etc.) and in terms of relational identities (i.e., doctor–patient, woman–woman, friend–friend, educator–student, partner–partner) and individual identities (i.e., practitioners and patients who are also wives, mothers, daughters, professionals, community members, etc.; for further interpretive descriptions of women and women's life experiences, see Kjernik & Martinson, 1986; Lewin & Oleson, 1985). By viewing health care encounters as social constructions, we widen our potential for understanding interactions between caregivers and patients as complex, multifaceted, and consequential.

Although our primary interest lies in the dyadic co-accomplishment of health care encounters, we pursue the dyad by recognizing that the individual participants—both the caregiver and the patient—enter the room as complicated, multidimensional people with preconceptions about how medical encounters "ought" to transpire, prior knowledge about each other and medical situations, and diverse and often contradictory goals. We avoid handling these individuals simplistically, monolithically, in terms of their identities and in terms of their goals for the encounter and for their relationship with each other. As detailed in Chapter 2, the chaos and fragmentation of the postmodern era precludes a shallow, singular depiction of the caregiver–patient relationship and of the participants who inherently co-create that relationship.

Because caregivers and their patients enter the examining room as social actors who *do* embrace sundry, often contrasting identities and goals and who *do* have a mix of conflicting preconceptions about what to do or how to proceed, each health care encounter requires each participant to carefully, artfully, attempt to understand the situation and the other's preferences for proceeding. In his writings on hermeneutics, Gadamer (1975, 1976, 1988) argued that interpretation constitutes an ongoing, emergent, temporal process. Given the vast range of options and influences in this postmodern era, caregivers and their patients must inherently struggle to attain a working consensus of "what is going on here," amidst the frustration of not being just in one place at once and not being constrained to simply one or another relational or individual identity. There is no longer just one way to interpret health care encounters nor singular, static, a priori identities and goals. At no previous time has the hermeneutic process been more difficult or more necessary than now, especially in the health care context.

Thus, throughout their brief exchanges, caregivers and patients face the challenge of making preferences for how encounters should ensue and for relational and individual identities and goals available to each other. In this volume, we explore how they do so, focusing on the co-accomplishment of communicative activities that work reflexively to enable the participants to display and respond to relational and individual identities and goals. For example, unlike cognitive approaches that treat constructs like goals as internal states (see Greene & Lindsey, 1989), our emphasis on goal work as an interactional accomplishment is consistent with other work on multiple goals from a discourse-based perspective (see Bavelas, 1991; Mandelbaum & Pomerantz, 1991; Sanders, 1991; Tracy, 1984, 1991a, 1991b; Tracy & Coupland, 1990). Like those other works, we focus on the micro-level, co-construction of goal work, treating it as emergent, temporal, and co-accomplished through conversation (see also Beck & Ragan, 1995; Ragan, Beck, & White, 1995; Smith-Dupre & Beck, 1996).

Through this micro-analytic, ethnomethodological approach to the social construction of aspects of women's health care encounters, we gain an appreciation for the interactional means through which women patients and their caregivers co-create their encounters and co-accomplish their relational and individual identities and goals by viewing what those participants have access to during their encounters—verbal and nonverbal behaviors. This ethnomethodological orientation to our data permits us to concentrate on otherwise taken-for-granted aspects of mundane conversation by making them problematic, forcing an exploration of how individuals, on the most local level, co-create intersubjective realities (see Garfinkel, 1967).

Although we describe potential influences on the achievement of activities during health care encounters later in this chapter, we heed the recommendation of Frankel (1989) and other ethnomethodologists that we should avoid a priori assumptions that all or any of those issues are salient for the participants. Instead, our analysis focuses on how the participants make such influences relevant in their interactions and on how those interactions permit or do not permit the participants to display and achieve their respective, preferred identities and goals for the encounter.

This micro-analytic approach to women's health care encounters enables us to abstain from the over-simplifying exercises of doctor bashing or advocating consumerism. Instead, based on more than 10 years of research on naturally occurring interactions between women and their caregivers as well as our own diverse experiences as patients who happen to be women (see Appendix A), we strive to move more productively toward identifying how participants in health care encounters can co-define at least a fragment of their relationship as a partnership and how they can attain a cornucopia of potentially contradictory relational, medical, and educational goals held by both participants—caregiver *and* patient.

INFLUENCES ON WOMEN'S HEALTH CARE

The need for such an interactional dynamic is especially critical in the context of women's health care encounters. Considerable research suggests that women patients have had problems with health care. It is important to emphasize that not all women experience problems with their health caregivers. Certainly, not all women have (or will) suffer because of inadequate information, insufficient preventative screenings, and inappropriate diagnoses and treatments. Admittedly, not all women and their caregivers co-construct an interactional dynamic where power plays a role. Perhaps the only influence that universally impacts all health care encounters (with women or with men patients) is the lack of available time in which to realize the multiplicity of possible identities and goals.

However, it is within this historical and social context (and amongst the glut of information—and potentially misinformation—about health care for women) that women come to encounters with their doctors. As we describe this context, we do so hesitantly, realizing that the incredible diversity of perspectives, reactions, and experiences (by both caregivers and patients) precludes specifying "a" reality. Yet, the following review offers a depiction of the complexity and paradoxes of the postmodern era—a virtual bombardment of information that contains no absolutes, echoes of voices of women who shout similar stories although no experience can be the same as another.

Hence, we begin by summarizing research from the medical community as a two-fold rationale for our focus on women and women's health. Women have not only suffered because of inadequate information, screenings, and treatments; women participate in interactions with their health caregivers amidst the paradox of wanting to trust their caregivers yet sorting through a wealth of information that indicates that perhaps they should not do so.

CENTRAL PROBLEMS FOR WOMEN PATIENTS

Although a general concern has emerged during the 1990s about the cost, quality, and availability of health care services for all U. S. citizens, women, in particular, face a health care system that often seems not to meet their needs. In the mid-1990s, some 35 years after women began their fight for quality and equitable treatment from the medical profession, women continue to confront problems on numerous levels, such as discrimination in medical research (Bennett, 1993; Charo, 1993; Council on Ethical and Judicial Affairs, the American Medical Association, 1991; Gorenberg & White, 1991–1992; Low, Joliceour, Colman, Stone, & Fleisher, 1994; Mastroianni, Faden, & Federman, 1994a, 1994b; Pfallin, 1994; Sechzer, Griffin, & Pfallin, 1994; Taylor, 1994) and discrimination in the availability of insurance and health care providers (Clancy & Massion, 1992; The Commonwealth Fund, 1993; Halvorson, 1993; Muller, 1992). However, in this age of increased awareness about women's health issues and about equality for women in other arenas, we are stunned that research reports suggest that women of the 1990s, like their sisters in the 1960s and before, still struggle to attain their medical, educational, and relational goals during their interactions with their health caregivers (Apple, 1990; Batt, 1994; Budoff, 1994; The Commonwealth Fund, 1993; Crook, 1995; Fee, 1982; Fisher, 1995; Friedman, 1994; Healy, 1991; Holmes & Purdy, 1992; Keyser, 1984; Laurence & Weinhouse, 1994; Nechas & Foley, 1994; Sherwin, 1992; Smith, 1992; Todd & Fisher, 1993; West, 1994).

We believe that women face difficulties in receiving care that are unique from their male counterparts. However, our goal here is not to bemoan discrimination but rather to provide a rationale for why women patients merit particular consideration. Although it is vogue to refer to a problem as a "crisis," we believe that the term aptly depicts the condition of health care for women in the United States. Research reports on serious voids in care for women in the United States have prompted a concerted effort by the National Institutes of Health to encourage research on women's health (LaRosa, 1994; Townsend, 1992) as well as numerous publications (Laurence & Wienhouse, 1994; Nechas & Foley, 1994) and episodes of television shows, such as *The Oprah Winfrey Show* ("How Medicine," 1994; "What Every Woman," 1993) and *Dateline NBC* (NBC News Transcripts, 1995), which tell how, case after case, women patients leave health care encounters with inadequate information, insufficient preventative screenings, and inappropriate diagnoses and treatments.

Women Patients Lack Information

Women need quality information more than ever about everything from protection from sexually transmitted diseases (STDs) to advice on wellness practices such as good nutrition, exercise programs, and reductions in smoking or alcohol or drug use. However, recent studies assert that such information does not tend to emerge during health care encounters. Information dissemination during patient interactions with OB-GYNs is a prime example of this problem. Although more than half of the women in the United States use their OB-GYNs as their primary physicians (ACOG News Release, 1993), a survey conducted for the American College of Obstetricians and Gynecologists (ACOG) indicates that few OB-GYNs offer counseling on STDs and HIV/AIDS (22%), osteoporosis (17%), drug abuse (13%), physical abuse (5%), diet and exercise (48%), medication use (43%), and mental health issues (14%). These figures are shocking, especially given the number of women who are impacted by these topics. For example, Galsworthy (1994) observed that 80% of the more than 25 million individuals in the United States who suffer from osteoporosis are women and that, ironically, "osteoporosis to a large extent is preventable and treatable" (p. 158).

One might excuse OB-GYNs for not spending time on issues that do not fall within their speciality area (setting aside, for the moment, the fact that women tend to rely on their OB-GYNs for primary care). However, the lack of information extends to areas that do directly impact reproductive care. Surprisingly, the survey found that only 31% of OB-GYNs even advise their patients about family planning and preconception care, despite the fact that these *are* reproductive issues, not simply primary care issues. Furthermore, although only 5% of the physicians responded that they talk about physical abuse with their patients, a recent study suggests that physical abuse occurs at an alarming rate during pregnancy and that this abuse results in babies who are more likely to be premature or underweight at birth, putting them at 40 times the risk of dying during their first month than other babies (ACOG News Release, 1996). Given that 60% of the pregnant women who indicated that they were abused also said that they lacked—yet desired—information about how to get help, the need for OB-GYNs to disseminate information on this topic is clear. As Dr. John R. Albert, the primary researcher, in the study and the associate director of maternal/fetal medicine in Carolinas Medical Center in Charlotte, North Carolina, asserted, "Pregnancy is a window of opportunity for physicians to improve the quality of life for their patients, since this may be the only time these abused women seek medical care" (ACOG News Release, 1996). Hence, the issue of physical abuse is relevant to the specific concerns of the OB-GYN, yet the issue is routinely not broached by caregivers and not disclosed by patients.

Another seemingly important topic for OB-GYNs to discuss with their patients was not even included on the survey of possible topics—cigarette smoking. However, as Townsend (1992) argued, "cigarette smoking remains the most important cause of preventable [infant] mortality and morbidity, yet women continue to smoke during pregnancy" (p. 158). The overall health threat for women who smoke makes this area even more significant. Lung cancer has emerged as a close second to breast cancer as the most prevalent form of cancer in women (Weisensee, 1986), and a 10-year study suggests that 54% of coronary heart disease in women may be attributed to smoking (Colditz, 1990; see also White, 1993).

Although public health campaigns may disseminate information on issues like smoking and STDs via the mass media, the accomplishment of patient education during interactions between caregivers and their patients localizes that information for patients, making both the risks and the opportunities for prevention more personal and perhaps more urgent. As the percentage of women who contract HIV/AIDS escalates (Bell, 1992), and the number of women who are diagnosed with syphillis rises to a 40-year high (Townsend, 1992), the need is clear for the accomplishment of interactional dynamics wherein education becomes a priority for both caregivers and patients. For instance, according to Townsend (1992), the rampant spread of STDs alone, largely due to the lack of understandable, accurate information, has resulted in "more than 100,000 infants [who] die or suffer with birth defects . . ." (pp. 205–206).

The fact that OB-GYNs are more or equally as likely to provide information to their patients as other types of doctors on all but three topics—diet and exercise, medication use, and mental health (ACOG, 1996)—makes the findings of the ACOG survey even more distressing. A study by the American Cancer Society (ACS) corroborates the ACOG survey results about the dissemination of information to women patients. According to the ACS study on physicians' attitudes and practices in early cancer detection (American Cancer Society, 1990), only 42% of OB-GYNs raise the subject of skin cancer with patients who exhibit no signs of sun-damaged skin, and even fewer (29%) warn patients about the dangers of exposure to the sun. As a result of the significant failure of caregivers to inform their patients about preventative practices and warning signs, the Commonwealth Fund Survey of Women's Health (The Commonwealth Fund, 1993) emphasized that the health risks to women are great (from heart disease, lung cancer, skin cancer, osteoporosis, STDs, etc.) because women "lack sufficient knowledge about how to protect themselves" (p. 6).

The irony in the forenoted studies is that women patients and their caregivers live in a time when individuals are literally bombarded with information on a daily basis. Media reports of medical research abound in newspapers, on television, and over the Internet. Warnings about cancer threats and STDs flood bulletin boards in schools, public transportation waiting areas, billboards on highways, even the sides of buses. Individuals who are not particularly seeking out information can readily stumble over it as they go about their daily lives.

However, profusion of information causes a cacophony of confusion. Patients get swept up in a virtual tidal pool of potentially conflicting facts, figures, reports, and recommendations. Certainly, a few patients may believe that they have answers and thus not feel the need to question; others may prefer to cope with illness or medical adversity by avoiding information (see Humphrey, Littlewood, & Kamps, 1992; McIntosh, 1976). However, more than ever before, patients do have questions and do want answers (see Hack, Degner, & Dyck, 1994). Not knowing how to ask or feeling uncomfortable about doing so, patients often refrain from questioning their doctors (see Beisecker & Beisecker, 1990; Frankel, 1990, 1995; Roter, 1979, 1984; Ten Have, 1991; Weijts, 1994; Weijts, Widdershoven, & Kok, 1991; Weijts, Widdershoven, Kok, & Tomlow, 1993; West, 1984, 1993; Wheeless, 1987; Young & Klingle, 1996).

As we discuss in more detail later in this chapter and in Chapters 2 and 3, patients must juxtapose a plethora of contradictory ideas about what they want to gain during the encounter mixed incongruently with their preconceptions about their caregivers and health care encounters in general. Especially for women patients in Western culture, expectations abound about what constitutes "appropriate" behavior in the presence of someone (such as a health caregiver) who has more knowledge and expertise than they do. At the most basic level, patients continuously—albeit unsuccessfully— attempt to reconcile the paradox of wanting (notably, to varying extents, depending on the specific patient) to get answers and to participate in decisions with the perception (and with some degree of trust) that the health caregiver has the knowledge and training to give information and to do what is necessary to define the problem and to offer solutions. For patients to attempt to direct the interaction by bringing up topics (thus, implicitly suggesting what their practitioners should consider or treat as relevant) or for patients to probe deeper into their practitioners' diagnoses or recommendations for treatments may seem, at least at some level, to implicitly call their practitioners' status as expert into question. To do so, the patients shift the nature of their relationships with practitioners away from a model that is socially and culturally familiar and comfortable to a model where they necessarily assume more responsibility.

Especially for women, this move to a more consumer-oriented, assertiveness-based model is not easily reconciled with the ways in which women are socialized to interact with others. Although a number of writers advance the astute caution that variables (such as race, education, sexual preference, and social class) interact with gender, making widespread generalizations difficult (see Gaines, 1995; Halberstadt & Saitta, 1987; Haraway, 1988; Harding, 1991; Huston & Schwartz, 1995; Kramarae, 1996; Spelman, 1988; West, 1993b; Wood, 1996), Tannen's (1994) review of the considerable research that has been conducted by gender communication researchers points to obvious differences in the ways in which males and females tend to interact (see also Tannen, 1990). The traditional socialization of women to a particular type of interactional role (such as nurturer, comforter, and supporter) has historically contributed to, and perhaps extended from, interactional differences between women and men. Such differences include the tendency of women to use more indirect talk and verbal fillers (Lakoff, 1975) and to use less verbal emphasis (Francis & Wales, 1994) than their male counterparts. Females also tend to interrupt men less than men interrupt women (West & Zimmerman, 1983; Zimmerman & West, 1975).

Hence, for women patients, "speaking up," particularly in a direct manner, during health care encounters entails overcoming cultural and social preferences for not doing so. It also requires them to just speak up in an interactional context where their questions may be treated by their caregivers as dispreferred, thus reinforcing their silence and passivity (Corea, 1977; Coulthard & Ashby, 1976; Davis, 1988a, 1988b, 1993; Davis & Fisher, 1993; Fee, 1982; Fisher, 1986, 1991, 1993a, 1993b, 1996; Lipsitt, 1982; Roberts, 1981; Todd, 1993; Todd & Fisher, 1993; Weaver & Garrett, 1982; Weijts, 1994; West, 1993a).

As we detail in Chapter 4, the art of patient education for both participants stems from the careful delineation of what to ask, how to ask, what to disclose, and how to ensure understanding. Patient education involves much more than simply "telling facts"; it necessitates facework on the behalf of patients who do not want to appear "stupid" and who may juggle the need to understand with the potential of insulting their caregivers with questions about explanations, recommendations, or even about contradictory information from other sources.

Patient education also requires facework on the behalf of caregivers who want to share information but who also want to treat their patients as knowledgeable. However, the gap in knowledge between caregivers and their patients makes the accomplishment of both of those simultaneous goals a challenge.

Although "just sharing the 'facts' " sounds simple, it is much more problematic for caregivers paradoxically because they do know so much more than their patients. Caregivers come to the encounter within the context of their own educational background, professional status, social status, personal experiences, and so on. Caregivers certainly interact in their everyday nonmedical lives with and like other nonmedical professionals. However, by necessity, the language that they learn in medical school is far different than that of everyday life—terms depict ideas, illnesses, and issues that nonmedical personnel do not need to know until they are directly impacted by them. The lack of shared language between caregivers and patients perpetuates the knowledge differential unless the caregiver becomes an artful translator or the patient learns the new language (see Thompson & Gillotti, 1993).

Even if caregivers can overcome the absence of a shared symbol system, no easy answers exist about what information, or how much information, to share with patients (see Katz, 1984; Maseide, 1981). Like their patients, caregivers wrestle with the swirling influx of information—both in their capacity as professionals and as people in the world. Scores of research reports fill medical journals and media reports; keeping up with the rapid current of information can be a full-time job, and sorting through the depths of those reports and determining relevance for individual patients can be overwhelming. The paradox for caregivers is realizing that their patients hunger for answers amidst all of the studies while recognizing that "an" answer may not yet be available and that time may preclude addressing all topics and all options.

Given their ever-changing, ever-emergent, multifaceted relationships with their patients, caregivers confront difficult choices about what issues to raise and what issues to table, given time constraints and the legion of possible topics and face considerations. As such, it is not surprising that a number of studies suggest that caregivers *do* sometimes fail to discern the extent to which patients desire information (Joos, Hickam, & Borders, 1993; Roter, 1983; Waitzkin, 1984) as well as what issues are important to patients (Barrett & Roberts, 1978; Goldberg, Guadagnoli, Silliman, & Glicksman, 1990).

However, regardless, and perhaps because, of the challenges of an over-abundance of information, confusing and conflicting cultural and role ex-pectations, and facework, the most pervasive problem, per the forenoted studies on the lack of information dissemination, has been the prevalence of silence (see Katz, 1984; for related argument, see also Roter, 1984, for research on patient question-asking and patient satisfaction). Crook (1995) gave the account of one patient, "Gilda," who experienced depression after giving birth. Gilda explained: "I couldn't really ask my doctor for help. I always felt like I would be a failure if I had to ask. But then, he could see I was in trouble and he never suggested any help. I didn't do anything and he didn't do anything." (p. 250). As Frankel and Beckman (1989) observed, the failure of caregivers and their patients to co-produce an interactional context in which patient concerns are voiced and addressed often results in a situation where patients ever so quietly listen to recommendations and then discard them as either not feasible or too costly in terms of financial expense, time, or personal sacrifice. By silently taking their own path (as opposed to sharing possible obstacles to actually accepting rec-ommendations with their caregivers), those patients do not benefit from a discussion of options, alternatives, and health ramifications of those choices. In Chapters 3 and 4, we strive to describe ways in which caregivers and patients may end their silence and begin an educational dialogue as partners.

Women Patients Lack Preventative Screenings

At a time when more diseases than even before are treatable and curable—if detected early (Thomas & Fick, 1994)—women need to be advised and encouraged to be screened for breast and cervical cancers. However, recent studies indicate that such screenings are simply not being done according to the ACS standards (Cohen, Halvorson & Gosselink, 1994; The Common-wealth Fund, 1993; Lurie et al., 1993; National Institutes of Health, 1996a, 1996b).

Lurie et al. (1993) found that less than half of the internists and family practitioners surveyed conducted Pap smears and breast examinations as recommended by the ACS standards. Whereas 80% of the OB-GYNs did test as recommended, notably 20% of the OB-GYNs did not. In a separate study, Majeroni et al. (1993) also discovered that less than half of both male and female doctors performed rectal examinations, mammograms, and Pap smears as recommended by the ACS, and only 55% did breast examinations. Perhaps the most shocking aspect of these findings was that by Lurie et al. (1993) regarding the group of doctors who rated the lowest for conducting screenings. Despite the increasing emphasis in medical school on the importance of pre-ventative care and early detection of disease, Lurie et al. (1993) reported that doctors under 38 years old tend to screen the least for these women's illnesses.

The lack of preventative screenings has dire consequences for women. According to a National Institutes of Health (NIH) Consensus Development Conference Statement on Cervical Cancer (National Institutes of Health, 1996a), more than half of the women who are diagnosed with invasive cervical cancer have never had a Pap smear, and another 10% of those women report that they did not have one in the 5 years prior to detection of the disease. Ironically, Dr. Allen Lichter, co-chair for the NIH panel, asserted, "If we could reach all of the women in this country who are not getting regular Pap tests, we could eradicate this form of cancer" (National Institutes of Health, 1996a).

However, the effort to increase preventative screenings cannot just "reach" women; it must include women as active participants. Caregivers cannot corral women, forcing them to come in for annual checkups, Pap smears, mammograms, and so on. Although caregivers have a responsibility to raise issues when they get the opportunity to talk with women patients (as dis-cussed in the previous section), women must participate in the dialogue. To do so, women patients must initiate the conversation by making critical appointments and by asking good questions when speaking with their doc-tors. The combination of a void of financial resources and good infor-mation as well as the perception of possible cultural barriers against seeking care—especially gynecological exams—thrust some women into a dangerous abyss of ignorance.

Research indicates that the problem intensifies for women who are the least likely to receive good health information—the elderly and lower income women (Fox, Sui, & Stein, 1994; Landen & Lampert, 1992; National Institutes of Health, 1996a). Fox et al. (1994) reported that "breast cancer screening rates, especially for mammography, continue to lag for older women, particularly for women older than 65 years old" (p. 2058). Furthermore, as panelists at the NIH Conference on Cervical Cancer observed, although 41% of cervical cancer deaths occur in women over age 65, 50% of women over age 60 wait more than 3 years between Pap smears (National Institutes of Health, 1996a). Landen and Lampert (1992) observed that the lack of screenings for cervical cancer among Native-American and Alaskan Native women has made cervical cancer a significant health problem for these populations.

The lack of emphasis on preventative screenings is even more disturbing, given that women's lives literally depend on detecting disease in the earliest possible phase (Austoker & Sharp, 1993; Thomas & Fick, 1994). For example, Thomas and Fick (1994) noted that "approximately one of every nine women will develop breast cancer by age 85" (p. 152). However, they also stressed that the 5-year survival rate for both in situ cancer of the breast and for in situ cervical cancer is 100%, if the disease is caught in its initial stages (Thomas & Fick, 1994). In the case of both of these diseases, lack of information and lack of screenings literally link together to cause unnecessary pain, suffering and death.

Laurence and Weinhouse (1994) told the story of Cass Brown, a 32-year-old woman. Although breast cancer is rare for women under 40, these women are not risk free. Despite this, Ms. Brown's doctor finished doing a pelvic exam and obtaining a Pap smear and asked her, "You don't need a breast exam, do you?" When she identified a lump above her breast a few weeks later, she had a mammogram that revealed a "highly suspicious mass." She not only suffered the pain of the mammogram and the fear of the lump; she faced the subsequent criticism of a surgeon who contended that she was "too young" for a mammogram and that she did not need a biopsy. After Brown insisted on a biopsy, the surgeon called her with the results. According to Laurence and Weinhouse (1994), "uncomfortable and embarrassed, he couldn't choke out the word *cancer*" (p. 116). Yet, the lump was indeed malignant. If not for her own personal persistence, Cass Brown's cancer would likely have gone undetected until it progressed too far for treatment.

Cass Brown's story attests to the need for patients to participate in their health care, to learn about the need for preventative screenings, to insist that they be conducted as necessary, but, as we observed earlier, patients often stay silent. We are not arguing that patients know more than their caregivers or that caregivers may not or should not be trusted or that caregivers may be incompetent. Although Cass was "right" to demand the screenings, the doctor was also "right," given his knowledge of odds, his professional experience, his concern for overuse, and unnecessary use, of radiation, and so on. We are suggesting that caregivers and patients must realize the urgent need for adequate preventative screenings and that both must actively engage each other in a conversation about necessary tests, the benefits and risks that may stem from such tests, and a timetable for conducting those tests.

Medicine is not an absolute science; it is much more similar to an art. Because we cannot speak in terms of certainties and absolutes in any realm of this postmodern era, even in the area of health care, we urge a turn to dialogue, discussion, and collaboration. However, for the conversation to begin, the silence must end. In the case of preventative screenings, the lives of women linger in the balance.

Women Patients Lack Appropriate Diagnoses and Treatments

It is ironic that in the 1990s, a time when women are respected professionals and public officials, women face the paradox of sorting through information that suggests that they may obtain inappropriate diagnoses and treatments simply because they are women. Women often struggle against a gender bias that has been intensified by the historical unwillingness of the medical community to include women in scientific studies, and by the lucrative nature of surgical procedures that can be rationalized, although not completely justified, as medically necessary.

A number of scholars point to the likelihood that caregivers too often disregard key symptoms as unimportant, stress-related, or insignificant "woman's complaints" (Keyser, 1984; Laurence & Weinhouse, 1994; Nechas & Foley, 1994). Especially in the case of heart disease, studies indicate that women are much less likely than men to be tested (Mark et al., 1994; Shaw et al., 1994) and that women are much more likely than their male counterparts to receive different and less adequate treatments (Aaronson, Schwartz, Goin, & Mancini, 1995; Legato, 1994; Mark et al., 1994; Maynard, Litwin, Martin, & Weaver, 1992; Petticrew, McKee, & Jones, 1993; Steingart & Wassertheil-Smoller, 1992). As Steingart and Wassertheil-Smoller (1992) stressed, "To date, virtually every aspect of CAD [cardio-artery disease] management in women from the initial evaluation of symptoms to diagnostic test performance to decisions about treatment has been marked by confusion and controversy" (p. 13). The result is that women face greater health consequences, ranging from multiple by-pass surgeries to death, than men who come to their caregivers with the same initial symptoms (Becker et al., 1994; Clarke, Gray, Keating, & Hampton, 1994; Healy, 1991; Khan et al., 1990; Lamas, Pashos, Normand, & McNeil, 1995).

Although biological differences between men and women are sometimes used to explain variation in treatments according to gender, in many cases, caregivers simply overlook glaring symptoms of heart disease because it has been traditionally considered to be a male disease by researchers and heart disease specialists (Altman, 1991; Laurence & Wienhouse, 1994; Nechas &

Foley, 1994). Statistics abound that prove this belief to be a misconception that costs women vital time and often, their lives. For example, Eaker et al. (1993) noted that cardiovascular disease is the leading cause of death and disability for women, claiming more lives than "cancer, accidents, and diabetes combined" (p. 1999).

Unfortunately, because doctors have not typically viewed heart disease as prevalent in their female patients, women patients may not be encouraged to be alert for warning signs of heart disease nor to practice preventative measures (such as quitting smoking, eating better, and exercising more consistently) to decrease their risk of heart disease (Brody, 1995; Pilote, 1994). According to Brody (1995), only 4% of women perceive heart disease to be a serious health threat, whereas more than 8 times that many (35%) may actually develop heart disease. Brody (1994) suggested that "for many years, American women thought they were relatively immune to heart disease, long the leading killer of American men" (p. 17). However, as Starr (1992) stressed, "women may be dying from a misconception" (p. 35).

In addition to errors in treating and preventing traditionally "male" afflictions such as heart disease, research indicates that caregivers tend to recommend and conduct many more surgical procedures on women than they do on men (Keyser, 1984; Kolata, 1993; Laurence & Weinhouse, 1994; Nechas & Foley, 1994; Smith, 1992; West, 1994). For example, according to the National Center for Health Statistics (1991), 23% of women will have an appendectomy, as compared with 12% of men, even though the risk of appendicitis for women is relatively the same as for their male counterparts (6.7% for women vs. 8.6% for men).

The tendency to conduct unnecessary surgeries on organs that are specific to women is even more dramatic (see Keyser, 1984; Laurence & Weinhouse, 1994). West (1994) asserted that 90% of hysterectomies are extreme treatments and are not warranted by the patients' conditions (see also Smith, 1992). As Kjerulff, Langenberg, and Guzinski (1993) observed, "the hysterectomy rate for the United States is twice that of England and Wales, and more than three times the rate for Norway and Sweden" (p. 106).

Doctors often build on patients' fears of cancer by stressing, especially to women who are beyond childbearing years, that the female reproductive system is unnecessary and, as such, total hysterectomies are encouraged (see Finck, 1986; Fisher, 1986; Laurence & Weinhouse, 1994; Smith, 1992; West, 1994). Removing healthy organs as a preventative measure inflicts a number of health consequences on potentially unwitting, trusting patients. Although these physicians refer to the threat of potential subsequent illness as the impetus for such surgeries, Finck (1986) maintained that "the magnitude of this fear and the actual percentage of cancerous degeneration of fibroids do not correlate" (p. 205).

Similarly, in the case of breast cancer, the prevalent philosophy until recently has been to remove the entire breast, thus, theoretically, reducing the risk of recurrence. However, Kolata (1993) argued, as do many others, that lumpectomies have been proven as effective as mastectomies. Although breast cancer advocates launched a successful campaign to reduce the number of radical mastectomies as an automatic response to a diagnosis of breast cancer (Batt, 1994; Hilts, 1995; Rinzler, 1993; Solomon, 1991), Steele, Winchester, Menck, and Murphy (1993) reported, that the rate of lumpectomies, not partial mastectomies, ranged only from 20.6% to 55% depending on the geographical region of the country.

The risk of unnecessary surgeries extends from the threat of life-threatening illnesses to childbirth situations. The advent of managed care has reduced the financial viability of optional surgeries, like some elective cesarean (c) sections. Yet, this form of child delivery is much more common in the United States than in other countries with comparable rates of successful births. The rate of c-section deliveries quadrupled in the 22-year period between 1970 (5.5% of all births, $n = 195,000$) and 1992 (23.6% of all births, $n = 921,000$; U.S. Bureau of Census,1994).

At least one study supports the claim (advanced by Finck, 1986; Keyser, 1984; Smith, 1992, and others) that monetary and time considerations may influence a physician's decision to perform a c-section. Haas, Udvarhelyi, and Epstein (1993) found that the provision of health insurance to lower income women did not generate an improvement in maternal health but that it was positively associated with an increase in c-sections for those women. The increased use of technology may also constitute a possible explanation for more c-sections (see Laurence & Weinhouse, 1994; Roberts, 1981). The combination of highly advanced fetal monitoring and the likelihood of lawsuits if something would happen to go wrong despite that monitoring produces a situation where doctors could see the more invasive way as being more prudent, where the slightest sign of a problem on the monitor could provide an impetus for insisting on surgery.

In her 1986 book, Sue Fisher discussed her experience as a well-educated, articulate woman who had spent 6 years researching women's health care prior to the discovery of an ovarian mass in her own body. Fisher (1986) reported that she knew that the doctors would urge her to get a total hysterectomy and that she knew enough to know that such a surgery was not necessarily required. Although she did win her interactional struggle to choose what would happen to her body on the operating table, Fisher noted that the doctor's warning that the mass could return lingered in her mind, despite her extensive understanding of the research in this area. Fisher observed that her case was rare because she took a stand for her medical preferences and that "repeatedly, while doing research in departments of reproductive and family medicine, I saw physicians recommend treatments, and patients, usually unquestioningly, accept them" (p. 3).

In Fisher's sentence, we see the problem—the lack of collaboration, the lack of a partnership dynamic. However, we contend that the problem may not be simplistically defined as a case of tyranny by "unreasonable" doctors.

The paradoxical struggle for caregivers ensues as they stumble into the snare of "both–and-ness," necessarily working toward simultaneous, seemingly contradictory goals and identities. Caregivers may legitimately assume that patients rely on their medical expertise in the resolution of health care concerns (see Joos, Hickam, & Borders, 1993; Phillips & Jones, 1991; Stone, 1979). However, given the relatively recent trend toward a more consumer-like orientation by patients, caregivers face the ambiguity of not knowing which patients want to participate in decision-making (Hack, Degner, & Dyck, 1994) and, if patients do, how they can do so without extensive information (see Arntson, 1989). Thus, the paradox emerges from caregiver efforts to serve as both experts *and* facilitators for patient decision-making (see related work on participative decision-making by Ballard-Reisch, 1990, 1993; Schain, 1990).

Patients clearly expect their health caregivers to be experts on medical procedures, illnesses, treatments, and the like, yet the imprecision of medicine does not permit talk in terms of certainties or absolutes. Caregivers face the challenge of communicating their own uncertainties and limitations while attempting to present themselves as trustworthy experts who do have some degree of command over medical understanding (see Calnan, 1984; Waitzkin, 1985; Wiener, Fagerhaugh, Strauss, & Suczek, 1980).

Caregivers must also balance their self-presentation as "experts" with their relative desire to involve patients in the decision-making process. If the "expert" has "the" answer, then what role can the patient legitimately assume (see Smith & Pettegrew, 1986)?

Caregivers are thus compelled to juxtapose competing, concurrent goals of enabling patients to participate in decision-making about procedures, tests, and treatment plans while retaining the ability to offer recommendations and to encourage that those recommendations be followed. Even caregivers who want their patients to participate actively in their own health care may feel strongly that they must persuade their patients to comply with specific courses of action (from quitting smoking or drug abuse to ending a physically abusive relationship to agreeing to an operation), especially in this era of litigation (for discussions of ethical and legal concerns with patient compliance, see Eraker, Kirscht, & Becker, 1984; Menken, 1992). Advocating a specific option while remaining open to input is difficult, particularly given the range of knowledge, understanding, and perspectives that caregivers and patients bring to their health care visits.

Thus, caregivers come to health care encounters with their own interpretations of the medical information and training that they have received and with their own diverse assortment of life experiences. Patients also enter the examining room with their own interpretations of health and health care, with scattered bits of knowledge about medical issues, with a multiplicity of possible, preferred relational and individual goals and identities. Arguably, both want the best outcome for the patient. However, as the literature on information dissemination, preventative screenings, and diagnoses and treatments for women suggest, 'best" is not a fixed entity to be achieved; one course of action is not always, absolutely, *the* way to proceed. As we stress throughout this book, partner-like decision-making between caregivers and patients facilitates the realization of the complex, multidimensional nature of caregivers and patients' identities and goals. Through such a dynamic, the expertise of caregivers and the knowledge and personal intuition of patients may be melded together in a joint effort for optimum health care.

However, the potentiality of such a dynamic is clouded by paradoxical influences. Reports such as the ones that are noted here contradict the "doctor-as-deity" myth. Caregivers do not have all of the answers; they do not always respond as patients would like; they cannot achieve unachievable perfection. Furthermore, despite calls for patients to participate, patients may feel constricted by perceived power differentials—to ask is to challenge, to challenge is to shatter an unspoken pane of glass that separates caregivers and patients.

PERCEIVED POWER DIFFERENTIAL IN HEALTH CARE ENCOUNTERS

The issue of power in health care encounters has been explored by a number of medical sociologists, health communication scholars, and feminists (see Calnan, 1984; Davis, 1985, 1988a, 1988b; Fisher, 1984, 1986, 1991, 1993a, 1993b, 1995; Mishler, 1984; Roberts, 1981; Shapiro et al., 1983; Silverman, 1987; Todd, 1989; Todd & Fisher, 1993; Waitzkin, 1985; West, 1994; Wiener, Fagerhaugh, Strauss, & Suczek, 1980). The traditional medical model, which until recently has been emphasized and implicitly advocated in medical schools across the country, positions the caregiver in a superior status to his or her patients (see Parsons, 1951). Although this model has been criticized and official medical school orientations toward the patient–practitioner relationship have shifted in favor of more participative models of medicine (see Wolinsky, 1980), in many cases, the institutional context of health care interactions still reflects and perpetuates a power differential between practitioners and patients, especially when the patients are women (Davis, 1985, 1988a, 1988b, 1993; Fee, 1982; Fisher, 1986, 1995; Fisher & Groce, 1985;

Katz, 1984; Todd, 1989, 1993; Treichler, Frankel, & Kramerae, 1984; West, 1984, 1993a).

Given our theoretical perspective that institutional power and structure are not imposed but rather are socially constructed by the participants (for related arguments on this micro-orientation to social structure, see Boden, 1994; Boden & Zimmerman, 1991; Davis, 1988a, 1988b; Drew & Heritage, 1992; Fisher, 1986, 1995; Helms, Anderson, Meehan, & Rawls, 1989), we suggest that power becomes manifested through the interaction between the participants. For example, the tendency of doctors to dominate discussions and to direct interactions by posing most of the questions is well documented (see Frankel, 1993a, 1995; West, 1993a; see also review by Modaff, 1995). Such interactional patterns contribute to a dynamic where the patient relinquishes her status as an active participant and becomes a passive object of medical attention (see Apple, 1990; Lewin & Olesen, 1985; Roberts, 1981).

Societal, cultural, and institutional expectations and perceived role obligations and constraints become realized and reified through the mundane ways in which the participants respectively contribute to the encounter. To contend that practitioners dictate interactions and that patients merely submit because of institutional roles that restrict their behavior is to dramatically oversimplify the underlying issues with which the participants must internally and interactionally negotiate.

A number of feminist critiques of women's health care point to the power differential between male caregivers, in particular, and their patients (see Corea, 1977; Davis, 1988a, 1988b, 1993; Davis & Fisher, 1993; Fee, 1982; Fisher, 1986, 1991, 1993a, 1993b, 1995; Todd & Fisher, 1993). Although we caution against global generalizations and sweeping conclusions, some preliminary studies do suggest some differences in male and female doctor interaction with patients (see Bensing, Brink-Muinen, & DeBakker, 1993; Brink-Muinen, DeBakker, & Bensing, 1994; Elstad, 1994; Ivins & Kent, 1993; Levinson, McCollum, & Kutner, 1984; Meewesen, Schaap, & Van Der Staak, 1991; Miles, 1991; Roter, Lipkin, & Korsgaard, 1991; Waller, 1988; Weisman, 1986; Weisman & Teitelbaum, 1985).

Notably, such research may reflect preconceptions rather than distinct behavioral differences. Given cultural expectations, women patients may visit female practitioners with the prior belief that female doctors will be different than male doctors (see Alexander & McCullough, 1981) and that, unlike their male counterparts, the female practitioners will engage in a similar interactional pattern as their women patients or be uniquely able to talk in terms of the lived experiences of female patients (see Allen, Gilchrist, Levinson, & Roter, 1993). At least two studies offer empirical support for a more symmetrical interaction between female doctors and their patients than between patients and male physicians described in other studies

(Smith-Dupre & Beck, 1996; West, 1984). Some scholars also point to nurse practitioners (who are typically female and who may be less likely than female physicians to be indoctrinated into a patriarchial model through medical school training) as offering a unique exception to the caregiver-dominant dynamic (see Beck & Ragan, 1995; Drass, 1988; Fisher, 1995; Ragan, Beck, & White, 1995).

Yet, it is imperative to remember that all health care practitioners are individuals, with their own personalities and styles of patient care. In the spirit of the fragmentation of the postmodern era, we believe that modernist tendencies to depict people as one way or another, especially in terms of gender stereotypes, provide a far too monolithic understanding of how, or why, people interrelate in particular ways.

Certainly, we do not discount the possibility that some women patients and their male caregivers may co-construct an interactional environment wherein caregivers may work to silence their patients, and patients may accept, or not dispute, that situational and relational definition (see Davis, 1988a, 1988b). As we detail in Chapter 2, however, the ways in which caregivers and patients verbally and nonverbally treat each other enable them to create and perpetuate interactional systems wherein dyadic systemic rules and roles are socially co-constructed; the interactants are not bound in terms of a priori institutional or gender constraints.

Differentials in levels of medical knowledge constitute an excellent example of how preconceptions manifest into behaviors and how behaviors reaffirm perceived power differentials. As caregivers serve as gatekeepers for patients, they inadvertently (yet inherently) widen the gulf between the worlds of caregivers and patients and, thus, perpetuate the perceived power differential (see Coleman, 1983; Shapiro, Najman, Chang, Keeping, Morrison, & Western, 1983). Building on the writing of Foucault (1979), Arney and Bergen (1983) asserted that "knowledge is power" and that "invoking knowledge about what is important to the person *is* the activity of power" (p. 5). In this case, a differential in medical knowledge can result in a perpetual cycle where the patient assumes her ignorance and remains silent and passive and where the caregiver, by default, chooses the topics which he or she believes to be relevant and offers recommendations based primarily on medical knowledge without the benefit of a complex understanding of the multifaceted patient before him or her, nor of the personal context in which medical decisions must be made.

INFLUENCE OF TIME CONSTRAINTS

Time impacts all health care encounters. The days of housecalls have transformed into day after day of filled waiting rooms and enormous time pressures for caregivers to attend to the most people in the least possible time—of course, while making the fewest possible mistakes. The economics of contemporary health care make this situation a stark reality for both caregivers and their patients. The rampant expansion of managed care and HMOs tighten the purses of possible insurance reimbursement for services to patients, compelling doctors to spend less time with patients (for related work, see Beck & Wilkens, 1996; Wilkens, 1996). As a result, caregivers may legitimately feel a need to "cut to the chase," and patients may feel a need to "not bother" their caregivers with "unimportant" information or to ask questions to clarify or to probe into practitioner recommendations.

Time constraints may hinder the ability—and, to varying extents, the willingness—of both participants to accomplish all of their relational, medical, and educational goals for the encounter. Within a tight time frame, the participants struggle to gain and disseminate information, assess medical conditions, make a diagnosis, discuss a course of action, and attend to relational needs. Furthermore, although health communication scholars continue to advocate a more participative orientation to health care encounters, frankly, participation demands dialogue that requires time.

PLAN OF THE BOOK

Researchers have thus far provided only partial pictures of communication during health care encounters, especially in light of the complexity and potential paradoxes of a multiplicity of confusing, contradictory influences on those encounters (such as reports of insufficient care of women—in terms of information dissemination, preventative screenings, and diagnoses and treatments—as well as real and perceived gender biases, time constraints, gaps in knowledge, perceived power or status differentials). Moreover, health care researchers have generally stopped short of treating caregivers and patients as multidimensional in terms of relational and individual identities and goals.

In our attempt to pursue the complexity of women's health care encounters, we advance a postmodern perspective of relational communication in the women's health care context. We believe that the issues with which female patients and their health caregivers continue to struggle are clearly relational ones: defining the multifaceted nature of the situation and their emergent relationship, co-creating and perpetuating a multiplicity of simultaneous, overlapping, often conflicting relational and individual identities, and discerning how they can *mutually* accomplish the many goals that they bring to the health care encounter.

This book responds to the needs of patients, practitioners, scholars, and health care educators to understand the relational dynamics that inherently underlie health care interactions between women and their caregivers. In particular, this data-based volume provides an innovative and important description—as well as useful exemplars—of how women's health care encounters may be constructed, how participants in the encounters assume and reify multiple relational and individual identities, and how relational, educational, and medical activities are co-accomplished by the participants.

This book extends from a program of research on women's health issues by the authors. More than 150 audiotaped, naturally occurring interactions between health caregivers and their female patients from three different health care settings (as well as ethnographic field notes in three additional settings that provide health care to women) constitute the data for this investigation. Chapters in this book explore the consequentiality of relational issues during women's health care encounters from a postmodern perspective and examine how health care participants co-accomplish relational goals as they work to co-define a plethora of relational and individual identities (Chapter 3), how those participants engage in activities that facilitate patient education (Chapter 4) and how those participants co-achieve activities related to medical care (Chapter 5).

Chapter 2 provides the reader with a background in relational communication theory; however, we move beyond traditional treatments of relational communication by taking a postmodern perspective. We believe that this perspective uniquely enables us to understand the health care encounter in light of the inherent complexity of the situation, the participants, and the relational dynamic between the participants.

Chapter 3 focuses on the interactional resources that can enable caregivers and patients to co-accomplish relational activities and, thus, to maintain and achieve their respective, preferred relational and individual identities during health care interactions. Chapters 4 and 5 move beyond the accomplishment of relational goals to explore how those relational activities facilitate the achievement of other critical goals, educational and medical. Chapter 4 identifies how attention to face management and other relational concerns enables practitioners to facilitate patient education and how the facilitation of patient education works, in turn, to enhance the relational and medical outcomes of the encounter. Chapter 5 examines the ways in which medical procedures can be introduced, explained and implemented as well as the ways in which medical information can be expediently obtained and disseminated. It also addresses how multiple goals may be achieved simultaneously (i.e., offering the type of explanation during procedures that leads to patient education and to patient participation in health care as opposed to just treating the patient's "problem").

Chapter 6 concludes the book by stressing how artful relational activities can be efficiently integrated into the encounter and how they can lead to subsequent improvements in a woman's health. The chapter emphasizes that relational activities empower women in our samples to participate more as partners in their health care because their caregivers tend to treat them as such.

The Consequentiality
of Relational Dynamics

"Amanda" sat on the edge of the examining table. The wait for the doctor to return to the tiny room had taken far longer than she had expected. She glanced around the room for something, anything, to read, hoping for some distraction from her nervousness about the unknown. The room was white and sterile, no magazines, no newspapers, no television, no noise, only the occasional rustle of the paper on the table when she shifted her weight. The silence itself was maddening. It left her alone with the nagging questions about her situation echoing through her mind. What could be wrong, she wondered? What could take so much time? What could possibly require this doctor to need to consult with someone else, and what did that mean anyway? Can I, should I, trust this person who I have never met before and yet with whom I've entrusted so much? She yearned for the sound of footsteps near her door in the hospital corridor.

Eventually, the doctor did return. He entered the room with two other men in white coats who wore hospital identification badges indicating their status as doctors. They said nothing. Amanda watched as they pulled out the stirrups and placed her bare feet in them. The only words that they spoke to her were "lay down and scoot back now." One after the other, they examined her. During their poking and probing and looking between her legs, they spoke to each other, using terms that Amanda had never heard before. But then, it seemed that she really shouldn't be hearing them now. In a surreal way, she felt like an eavesdropper, an intruder, on a conversation that was about her yet was not meant at all to include her. After the third doctor finished, the first doctor said, "We're through now," and the three left the room.

Alone in the silence again, Amanda wiped herself off. Her hands were shaking, and tears welled up in her eyes. She knew no more about her condition than she did before the men came into the room; however, she felt much more. In her mind, they had done as much as rape her. They had dismissed her, demeaned her, disregarded her status as a patient, as a participant, as a person.

She had entered the hospital on the recommendation of another doctor at a convenience clinic. She visited that doctor to get medication for what she had self-diagnosed as an ulcer. She had been under a lot of stress at work, and she was a newlywed of two months. She had told the doctor that her stomach was throbbing and that it was hard to stand up straight. During her questioning about Amanda's medical history, the doctor had learned that Amanda had irregular periods, and, because Amanda could not specify her last cycle, the doctor ordered a pregnancy test. To Amanda's surprise, it came back positive, and the doctor referred her to the hospital for testing to determine the source of her pain.

Amanda walked into the hospital feeling trepidation about the unexpected pregnancy and a range of other issues as well. Ironically, the only other pelvic exam that she had ever had prior to her experience with the three doctors was when she visited a nurse practitioner at a college health care facility to get birth control pills before getting married. She had avoided seeking gynecologic care during her adult life. Amanda found the entire idea of exposing herself to total strangers in the necessary way during pelvic exams to be reprehensible, and, upon admission to the hospital, she felt emotionally unprepared to handle the medical aspects of pregnancy (such as the need for pelvic exams), much less a pregnancy that seemed destined to be laden with complications from the very beginning.

After the doctors departed from the room, Amanda still lacked answers about what could be causing the pain. She did not obtain additional information about the status of the pregnancy nor guidance about her choices with regard to the pregnancy. She did not receive reassurance nor acknowledgment from any of the doctors that the situation was awkward and embarrassing. In fact, the doctors did not afford her any interactional opening where she could tell them about her concerns and fears. She only gained affirmation for what she had anticipated—pelvics hurt and make patients feel like mere objects on which to be acted.

Amanda climbed down from the table where she had sat for so long, reached for her clothes, and realized that she had never before felt such little control over her life and her health. Confusion, fear, humiliation, and now outrage stirred a new frenzy of questions that darted around inside her mind as she dressed and as she once more faced the agonizing silence of the tiny, white room.

This true story exemplifies health care encounters at their very worst—the doctors failing to at least acknowledge the patient and her needs and the patient failing to assert herself to voice those needs. Although some may argue that the problem in this encounter was a lack of communication, we suggest that the participants were very much engaged in communicative activities. For example, the doctors' lack of eye contact with Amanda, their lack of verbal interaction with her before, during, and after the examination, and their talk with each other as cohorts who share an exclusive language of medical jargon implicitly indicated (whether intentionally or not) their preferences for how the encounter should ensue, for their role in that encounter, and for the nature of their relationship with Amanda during the encounter. Amanda's silence and compliance with their directives worked to reify the doctors' definition of the encounter and their respective roles in the encounter.

The doctors and the patient in this example behaved in a manner that co-produced an encounter that was not patient-centered and that was not conducive to the accomplishment of educational and relational goals. Yet, through their mundane behaviors and nonbehaviors, spoken as well as unspoken words, they *did* communicate, and they *did* participate in relational communication.

This chapter details our stance that interactants cannot *not* communicate relationally. That is, they engage in the continual, although not necessarily conscious, process of positioning themselves in relation to each other through their verbal and nonverbal behaviors. This process of relational definition constitutes an ongoing, socially constructed, multifaceted accomplishment by interactants on at least the dyadic level. In this chapter, we briefly outline the major theoretical assumptions of this view of interpersonal communication through a review of the work by Gregory Bateson and the Palo Alto Group. We then summarize how those premises of relational communication have been applied to the health care context in earlier research. However, in light of our commitment to examining health care interactions as complex and often paradoxical exchanges between individuals with multiple possible goals, we move beyond the focus on relational control that is prevalent in the relational communication literature by suggesting a postmodern perspective of relational communication in health care encounters. We conclude the chapter by discussing the consequentiality of relational activities in light of this view of women's health care interactions.

RESEARCH ON RELATIONAL COMMUNICATION IN HEALTH CARE ENCOUNTERS

In an attempt to understand human relationships and to pinpoint problems in those relationships, it is easy to cast blame on one of the parties involved. In the case of health caregiver–patient relationships, caregivers may receive the blame for failing to educate or to communicate with their patients.

Patients may be criticized for their lack of assertiveness or unquestioning compliance with medical recommendations. The critical shortcoming of this individualistic approach to diagnosing the problems with health care encounters stems from the implicit disregard for the relational dynamic that emerges from the interaction; it discounts the importance of what occurs between, and gets co-constructed by, the participants.

Strongly influenced by general systems theory and cybernetics, Bateson (1935, 1951, 1958, 1972, 1979) laid the foundation for the relational approach to interpersonal communication, an approach that treats communication as processual and interactional rather than linear and individual. By viewing interactants as interdependent on each other, Bateson (1951) suggested that participants in a conversation co-create a system in which their verbal and nonverbal behaviors are consequential for how the interaction will ensue as well as for how they mutually co-define the nature of their relationship.

Borrowing from general systems theory then, Bateson and other scholars (especially those in the Palo Alto Group—see review by Wilder, 1979) who advocate this relational approach to interpersonal communication argue that the relationship between interactants constitutes an emergent dynamic that is inherently different from—and more than—the individual participants who are involved in that relationship (see Rogers, 1989; Rogers & Bagarozzi, 1983; Rogers & Millar, 1988; Watzlawick, Bavelas, & Jackson, 1967; Wilder-Mott, 1981; Wilder-Mott & Weakland, 1981). The relationship, as a system, must be conceptualized in terms of its wholeness and its nonsummativity (Watzlawick et al. 1967). Thus, by extension to the health care context, an analysis of *either* the health caregiver's *or* the patient's contributions to the interaction (or of either party's perceptions of the interaction) ignores the jointly co-constructed relationship between, and involving *both*, participants in the health care encounter.

Just as relationships cannot be appreciated by separating and analyzing individual system members, even single messages that are produced by those system members cannot be understood in isolation. The sequential nature of conversation underlies the consequentiality of messages. Prior turns at talk impact and constrain subsequent turns at talk; earlier actions (from nonverbal behaviors to episodes of silence to choices of activities) flavor the context within which next actions may be interpreted and then acted on by other interactants (see Bateson, 1951, 1972, 1979; Schegloff & Sacks, 1973; Watzlawick et al., 1967).

Watzlawick et al. (1967) and Goffman (1967) argued that "moves" in a conversation (i.e., turns at talk) resemble "moves" in a chess game. The continual limiting of "next moves" enables interactants to reflexively signal to each other an aligned orientation to conversational actions; that is, the reflexivity of language—both verbal and nonverbal—permits multiple meanings and communicative activities to be achieved simultaneously (i.e., the words and behaviors have their own meanings while also contributing to the emergent co-construction of local conversational activities—such as storytelling—see Garfinkel, 1967). As Cicourel (1970) explained, the reflexive nature of language allows interactants to guide subsequent behavior and to respond appropriately within the interactional context:

> The interpretive procedures and their reflexive features provide continuous instructions to participants such that members can be said to be programming each others' actions as the scene unfolds. . . . the participants' interpretive procedures and reflexive features become instructions by processing the behavioral scene of appearances, physical movements, objects, gestures, sounds, etc. into inferences that permit action. (p. 152)

For example, Beck (1994) detailed interactant orientation to the collaborated telling of a story. The co-constructed extended turn afforded to the teller indicated the orientation of the interactants to the co-production of conversation as the conversational action of storytelling constrained the possible, appropriate next utterances by interactants. As Schegloff (1982) explained, ". . . the production of a spate of talk by one speaker is something which involves collaboration with the other parties present, and that collaboration is interactive in character" (p. 73). Verbal and nonverbal cues or directions (possible because of the *both–and-ness*, the reflexivity, which is inherent to language) facilitate ongoing collaborations between interactants about what may legitimately take place next in conversations (see Beach, 1995; Beck, 1994, 1995, 1996; Heritage, 1984; Mandlebaum, 1990; Pomerantz, 1989, 1990; Sacks, 1984; Sacks, Schegloff, & Jefferson, 1974; Schegloff, 1982, 1986; Zimmerman, 1988).

Furthermore, Bateson (1935, 1951, 1958) insightfully alluded to the reflexivity of language with his observation that interactants accomplish more through their verbal and nonverbal behaviors than merely an exchange of information about some topic. Through their conversation and through the way in which they interact with each other, interactants also position themselves in relation to each other (see Duncan, 1967). Bateson (1951) explained that messages implicitly contain two components—a *report* or informational aspect and a *command* or relational aspect. The duality of messages enables interactants to offer and to receive, and confirm or disconfirm, content information as well as relational information (Bateson, 1951, 1972; Watzlawick et al., 1967; see also Cissna & Sieburg, 1981; Millar & Rogers, 1976; Parks, 1977; Rogers, 1981, 1989 as well as related arguments in sociolinguistics—Gumperz, 1971; Hymes, 1972—and in cognitive anthropology—Cicourel, 1970).

For example, Bateson's conception of symmetrical and complementary communication reflects this view that communication is inherently relational and reflexive (Bateson, 1935; see also Millar & Rogers, 1976; Parks, 1977; Rogers, 1981, 1989; Rogers & Bagarozzi, 1983; Rogers & Millar, 1988; Watzlawick et al., 1967). In a symmetrical communication pattern, the participants' behaviors mirror each other in terms of structure (e.g., assertion–assertion); in a complementary communication pattern, the participants' behaviors differ structurally (e.g., assertion–acceptance, question–answer). In a symmetrical relationship, both individuals assert control (except in the case of submissive symmetry where both individuals relinquish control), and, in a complementary relationship, one person asserts control while the other person accepts the first person's assertion. The patterns that emerge over time work to reify and reflect the nature of the relationship between the interactants as well as their respective roles in that relationship (see Bateson, 1979; Watzlawick et al., 1967; Rogers, 1981, 1989; Rogers & Millar, 1988). As Rogers (1981) emphasized, "Relational communication stresses the co-defining nature of relationships, the reciprocally defined rules of interdependence of system members" (p. 233).

The key here is that this process of mutual relational and role definition is ongoing and emergent. Given the interdependence of system members and the consequentiality of messages, Watzlawick et al. (1967) argued that interactants continually, although not necessarily consciously, engage in the process of maintaining or changing the nature of their relationship. As interactants respond (and even as they do not overtly or directly respond), they provide feedback about the status of the relationship and their treatment of each other as participants in that relationship (Watzlawick et al., 1967).

The reflexivity of language provides interactants with a means through which to co-determine and co-display their orientation to relational dynamics as well as, at the same time, to a multiplicity of social activities, such as discerning the meaning of messages, achieving a conversation, advancing situational definitions and individual identities (for related arguments, see also Beck, 1995; Cicourel, 1970, 1980; Frankel, 1984; Garfinkel, 1967). Such activities include the constant process of co-defining "how things work here" and "who are we in relation to each other" (see also writings by Goffman, 1959, 1967; Katovich, 1986, on self-presentation and identity).

Bateson's work (and later the efforts of the Palo Alto Group) provides the theoretical underpinnings for research in interpersonal communication that pursues the nature of the *interaction* (as opposed to the individual characteristics of the *interactants*) and that examines language as reflexive (as opposed to restricted to merely content information) (for other more indepth reviews of the evolution of the relational approach to interpersonal communication, see Parks, 1977; Rogers, 1989; Rogers & Millar, 1988; Watzlawick et al., 1967; Wilder, 1979; Wilder-Mott & Weakland, 1981). As such, it offers a foundation for work that pursues the co-constructed relational dynamic between participants.

Unfortunately, much of the research that acknowledges a theoretical debt to the original works by Bateson and the Palo Alto Group has taken a monolithic, albeit emergent, view of relationships and relational definitions, implying that dyads collaboratively create, maintain, and perhaps, change "a" relational definition to another one as the relational system evolves. Most of the research on relational communication patterns fails to recognize that dyads may struggle to reconcile multiple, simultaneous, and potentially contradictory relational definitions as well as overlapping, and contradictory, relational systemic boundaries and rules. Although Bateson (1955, 1972) and others (such as Watzlawick et al., 1967; see review in Wilder & Collins, 1994) discussed interactional paradoxes, none have advanced those writings by pursuing paradoxes that surface from diverse yet concurrent relational definitions. In fact, the primary empirical extension of work on relational communication has focused narrowly on the issue of relational control.

In particular, scholars have attempted to operationalize the concepts of *symmetry* and *complementarity* through various adaptations of relational coding schemes and have examined what kinds of communicative control patterns exist in relationships, such as family relationships (see Courtright, Millar, & Rogers, 1983; Ericson & Rogers, 1973; Millar & Rogers, 1976; Millar, Rogers, & Bavelas, 1984; Rogers, 1981, 1989; Rogers & Bagarozzi, 1983; Rogers & Farace, 1975; Rogers & Millar, 1988; Sluzki & Beavin, 1965). Research that recognizes the tradition of Bateson and the Palo Alto Group in the health care context also reflects a singularity in focus on relational control (Bermosk & Porter, 1979; McNeilis & Thompson, 1995; McNeilis, Thompson, & O'Hair, 1995; O'Hair, 1989; von Friederichs-Fitzwater, Callahan, Flynn, & Williams, 1991; for a review of literature on relational communication in the health care context, see Kreps, 1993).

Even if we put aside methodological concerns about coding schemes that are typically employed to assess relational control (see Emmert, 1989; Folger & Poole, 1982; Trenholm, 1991), the problem with this research is that it captures only a one-dimensional depiction of the relationship instead of treating the relationship (and the relational communication that occurs between the participants in the relationship) as a complex, multifaceted accomplishment (see Wilder, 1979). In the case of interactions between caregivers and their women patients, the emergent relationships are particularly complicated.

Women patients are not just individuals with health care concerns. They are daughters or mothers or wives with families and potentially multigenerational family responsibilities, professionals with career goals and organizational obligations, people with dreams, hopes, and fears, and consumers with economic concerns and constraints, and desires for choice and information. Women patients face the challenge of recognizing and communicating their need to seek medical expertise (thus acknowledging their own lack of expertise in this area) with their concurrent need to decide what will happen to their own bodies (and, in so doing, invoking their own knowledge of their bodies, life situations, and personal preferences) as they interact with their caregivers. For women patients, the complexity of the health care encounter extends far beyond the multiplicity of their everyday life roles; it involves multiple (and potentially paradoxical) relational, medical, and educational goals for their health care visits and for their interactions and relationships with health care providers.

Their caregivers are also not simply *caregivers;* they are professionals in a field where they confront the perception of having "the answers" and the reality that they may have mostly questions. Like their patients, they juggle their role in the health care encounter with their multiple family roles and responsibilities, organizational commitments, and personal dreams. Like their patients, they face interactional and relational paradoxes, such as the need to respond as experts and the need to offer choices to their patients.

When brought together during health care encounters, caregivers and patients necessarily struggle with co-determining what aspects of their lives and themselves should be relevant in the 10-minute visit as well as what dimensions of their multifaceted relationship should be emphasized at any given time during that visit. Although their relationship certainly involves their co-definition of their identity as "caregiver–patient," that identity may meld with other co-existing relational identities, such as "fellow women," "fellow mothers or wives or daughters," "fellow community members" and perhaps even "friends" and, hopefully "partners." The following interaction between a female doctor (D) and her patient (P) constitutes a perhaps unusual exemplar of the multiplicity of intermingled relational and individual identities that are possible beyond a strict conceptualization of the participants as "caregiver" and "patient."

Excerpt 1:

→ 1	D:	You're here for this to be your annual Pap, huh?
→ 2	P:	Unhum
3	D:	Okay. How's school going. You on break?
4	P:	It was last week.
5	D:	Okay
6	P:	Yeah back to classes again . . .
7		Yeah, I'm getting all my transcripts. I'm just gonna take
8		a couple of classes this summer. I'm gonna take non-
9		medical classes.
10	D:	Oh
11	P:	I'm taking a sociology class and I take, I take a couple
12		of psych classes and I want to take some art classes.
13	D:	Yeah that'll be good

14	P:	I'm taking things that have nothing to do with what I do.
15	D:	(laugh) When are you through, then, next year?
16	P:	Umhmm, yeah. I got seven more weeks of this year, then
17		next year, and then I'll be finished.
18	D:	Are you working this summer?
19	P:	I had asked to work here but they said my application was
20		too late.
21	D:	Oh oh
22	P:	And my work, when they sent the list downtown, I wasn't
23		on the list.
24	D:	Oh
25	P:	I guess my application was just too late.
26	D:	That's a shame.
27	P:	I didn't know if it would do any good to talk to (name of
28		official) or not.
29	D:	I'd talk to her.
30	P:	(illegible)
31	D:	Talk to her
32	P:	Cause I talked to her once, and she said yeah yeah do it,
33		and then I I said well, I could do personnel and with
34		people on vacation and whatever like that and a
35	D:	yeah oh yeah
36	P:	(unclear but something to the effect that the application
37		was late)
38	D:	It's my problem. I don't have enough time... I like to
39		teach
40	P:	yeah
41	D:	patients and all (.) You get a lot of good experience
42		teaching patients.
43	P:	yeah
→ 44	D:	[okay let you] hop right up here.
45	P:	[I don't know]
46	D:	organizing trying to organize our patient education
47		pamphlets and get them to the appropriate people. It
48		would help Cathcrine and Lora cause usually they're so
49		busy.
50	P:	umhum
51	D:	They don't have time to do much teaching . . . In fact, we
52		had a department head meeting yesterday where she
53		talked about she wanted the nursing staff to do more
54		teaching. So I would go to her.
55	P:	Yeah, it's hard when I know how busy you are. I know
56		it's not a slack time, usually it's feast or famine

```
  57           here.
  58    D:     I know (both laughing)
[87 lines later in same interaction]
→ 145  D:     Okay you still got a little discharge
→ 146  P:     well, sometimes, like the last few days it's like brown.
→ 147  D:     yeah
→ 148: P:     it comes down for a day or two
→ 149  D:     yeah . . . Okay now we take the speculum out now. Do you
  150          nurses learn how to do pelvic exams, as nurses?
  151   P:     We didn't get to do any, but we did learn it from the
  152          book.
  153   D:     Oh, I think you should. I like it. You know, I
  154          believe, I believe, I don't know, I believe that nurses
  155          have so much training that they should utilize it more.
  156   P:     umhum
  157   D:     I think that nurses can do normal prenatal care. I
  158          don't think that, you know, I think that's their
  159          training, and they can do Pap smears. What's the big
  160          deal?
  161   P:     Well, you know, we have to learn all theory and all of
  162          that—
  163   D:     —okay then why not
  164   P:     If we decided to be an OB nurse—
  165   D:     —yeah—
  166   P:     —we need to know how to do all those things, but we
  167          never get to do them as students.
→ 168  D:     Yeah, so I think you should be able to. There's your
→ 169          uterus, and it feels normal. No pain at all?
→ 170  P:     just a little bit
→ 171  D:     Yeah, it's not comfortable.
```

In Excerpt 1, the caregiver and patient co-produce an interactional environment wherein both parties permit dimensions of their selves to surface that may have been ignored in other health care encounters. They certainly could have focused talk and actions on the medical accomplishment of the Pap smear. Instead, here, they are not merely a doctor conducting and a patient complying with a particular medical task.

The caregiver refers to interests in ideas and issues beyond medical concerns; she positions herself as a fellow health care professional and, during other parts of the transcript, a mentor. The caregiver also facilitates the marking of the patient as also more than "just a patient" or even "just a student." She treats the patient as a potential co-worker and a future colleague. Furthermore, as a medical doctor, the caregiver voices respect for nursing (the patient's future occupation), integrating meta-references to mutual knowledge about nursing and the training of nurses throughout the examination. The caregiver offers encouragement and acceptance for the prospective nurse's choice of vocation.

Although they are in the middle of an uncomfortable and potentially face-threatening examination (see Beck & Ragan, 1992, 1995; Emerson, 1970; Ragan, 1990; Ragan, Beck, & White, 1995; Ragan & Glenn, 1990; Ragan & Pagano, 1987), this caregiver and patient float amidst sundry fragments of their individual identities (i.e., student, patient, caregiver, medical professional, and their relational identities (i.e., patient–caregiver, doctor–nurse, co-worker–co-worker, fellow women, fellow students). They do not take a rigid, modernist stance by positioning themselves as "either–or," (i.e., by saying "we are this now" or "we are that now"). They do not brush bits of their respective and collective identities aside in favor of a strict illumination of the caregiver–patient aspect of what evolves as a truly multifaceted relational dynamic.

Notably, caregivers will not always visit with patients who they know, nor will all patients have formal medical training before walking in the door. However, *all* patients and caregivers are more than just people who happen to enact those medical roles. Although medical work must (and, in this case, does) get done (see lines 1, 2, 44, 145–149, 168–171), this caregiver and patient give much more than simply a cursory wave to themselves and each other as multidimensional people, not just their status as "caregiver" or "patient." They seem to demonstrate an appreciation for the blur of intertangled identities.

The complexity that is inherent to health care encounters precludes a simplistic explanation or singularity in terms of role or relational definition. Mishler (1984) argued that more doctors should be concerned with the patient's "lifeworld" and suggests that interactants wrestle with a dialectical tension between talk of the "social" and of the "medical" worlds during medical visits (see also Clark & Mishler, 1992). We agree with Mishler that patients should be viewed in light of their lifeworlds; however, we believe that the multiple identities of both caregivers and patients are much more intertwined than this dichotomy implies. Furthermore, the stress on the patient's lifeworld ignores the multiplicity of identities that the doctor inherently brings to the encounter, and more importantly, it treats the emergent relational dynamic between caregivers and patients, their co-created, multifaceted relational identity, as insignificant. In the spirit of the postmodern era, we maintain that caregivers and patients may not be restricted to either one role or another nor may their relationship be limited to only one relational definition (and set of goals and systemic rules) as opposed to another; instead, a both–and view of relational dynamics in the health care context facilitates an appreciation for the multiple identities and realities with which caregivers and patients attempt to reconcile during their interactions.

A POSTMODERN PERSPECTIVE OF RELATIONAL
COMMUNICATION IN HEALTH CARE ENCOUNTERS

In his 1991 book, Gergen credited the explosive advent of technology and availability of information with the virtual implosion of the individual, the ultimate splintering of the traditional modernist conception of self. Thrust into the eddy of diverse images and perspectives that constantly swirls around them via the media and expanded interactional opportunities with others, individuals in the postmodern era paddle through turbulent currents from ideas to other ideas, relationships to other relationships, identities to other identities. Although they may periodically grasp a tree limb from the shore, they inevitably break away, only to continue their journey through their chaotic rivers of consciousness. However, even this image oversimplifies the chaos; individuals do not leave one idea, relationship, or identity and move on to the next. Postmodern living permits the ultimate both–and experience—individuals may dabble in a multiplicity of realities with a multiplicity of identities. As Gergen (1991) observed, "Our range of social participation is expanding exponentially. As we absorb the views, values, and visions of others, and live out the multiple plots in which we are enmeshed, we enter a postmodern consciousness" (p. 15).

Yet the blurred abundance of disparate possibilities, viewpoints, and relationships comes at the price of simplicity, clarity, and definitive expectations and definitions. Although life may never have been simple or easy before postmodernism, monolithic depictions of modern living on the mass media and from individuals' narrow circles of friends indicated that it should be. As one elderly character in the movie *Tootsie* contended, there once was a time when "men were men." In that time, before the onslaught of contradictory messages and alternative realities, there was a "right" way to be a "real" man, a "real" mother, even a "real" doctor, a "good" patient. Although families in everyday life have never been just like the Cleavers on television and doctor–patient interactions do not always result in positive outcomes nor satisfied patients ala Marcus Welby, the myth of certainty and objectivity constitutes a staple of modernism, people pursuing "a" truth, "a" right way of being, behaving, and believing.

As Pollner (1987) explained, "The assumption of an 'out there,' 'public,' or 'objective' world is a central feature of a network of beliefs about reality, self and others . . ." (p. ix). For example, each time health care participants attempt to "play by the rules" or assume "authority," they do so by relying on and taking for granted the assumption of "a" structure that constrains interactant behavior (Collins, 1981a, 1981b; Garfinkel, 1967; Hilbert, 1990; Pollner, 1987; Schutz, 1962; Zimmerman & Pollner, 1970). Despite the fleeting efforts of social actors in everyday life to find and link on to something stable "out there somewhere somehow," consistent with postmodernists, ethnomethodologists suggest that those social actors can actually only try to perpetuate their lay perspectives of "a" structure, "a" reality, "a" set of rules and roles—by simply acting as though structure, reality, and rules stand external to the interaction (see Cicourel, 1968, 1970; Collins, 1981a, 1981b, 1987; Garfinkel, 1956, 1967; Heritage, 1984; Knorr-Cetina, 1981; Manning, 1970; McHugh, 1968; Pollner, 1987; Schegloff, 1987; Turner, 1985; Wilson, 1970). They are destined to dart around perpetual mazes, trying to locate "the" right path despite the overwhelming number of frustrating options, trying to attain the unattainable, trying to keep their worlds from continually spinning and mixing up the possibilities, trying to end their frazzled search for scripts, clarity, and absolutism.

In postmodernism, individuals face the ongoing struggle to understand and construct their fragmented selves and relationships while bombarded by unceasing waves of scattered and contrasting bits of information from the media and their many interactional partners about what relationships should be like, about how people should treat each other in situations that lack simplistic definitions (yet paradoxically that may seem pre-scripted by rigid institutional definitions), about what their roles should even entail, and so on—such as how doctors should care for patients and how patients should respond to doctors (for related articles on role expectations for physicians and patients, see Cichon & Masterson, 1993; Krulewitch, 1980). The postmodern dilemma stems from the irreconcilability of those wisps of insight. The multiplicity of perspectives defy packaging into neat, clean, clear definitions about what constitutes a particular type of person or role behavior.

As Gergen (1991) suggested, the ability to defy geographical boundaries by expanding networks of potential interactional partners far beyond a very localized community and to skip through a vast array of data and ideas has not unveiled one objective truth or one accepted way of being or proceeding. The endless sifting through the multiplicity of vistas contributes to quite the contrary conclusion. Even in the case of information about something that is not social, relational, or driven by human interactions, such as scientific studies, one truth eludes us. For example, reports of research on illnesses, drugs, and preventive health abound, yet the results are often contradictory and lack specificity and certainty. The frantic search for answers and truth has unturned only perspectives, even in a scientific and heavily institutionalized field such as medicine.

The absence of one way of acting or proceeding obscures decisions about how to interact with others, especially in institutionalized settings. Yesterday, the roles of "doctor" and "patient" seemed set; today, interactants tentatively assume those roles amidst ambiguity. Although the framing of doctors as "empowerers" and patients as "consumers" may sound enticing, they are difficult to put into practice because no clear definitions exist about how one empowers or consumes in the "right" way within this particular context, a context where the remnants of rigid, albeit perceived, institutional roles continue to lurk in the examining room.

Patients may receive tips from friends, read articles in the popular press, or engage in dialogues with people on the Internet or in support groups about how to be a good patient, how to be a good health care consumer, how to handle a medical concern, and so on (see e.g., Duck, 1992; Sharf, 1988; Tardy, 1994). However, the complexity for patients lies in discerning how to fit the pieces of advice together when those pieces come from not one but many different, often contradictory perspectives on how patients should interact with their doctors and on how goals may be best achieved. For example, hesitant because of mixed messages from media reports or well-meaning friends about health caregiver motivations for recommending tests or procedures, patients may want to appear well-informed so they do not get "ripped off" by their health caregivers. The paradox results from the concurrent desire to gain information from their health care providers, thus, demonstrating some degree of trust in the providers' respective ability to give that information. Furthermore, patients may want to be assertive and strong yet they likely want to do so in a manner that will not be offensive or threatening to their health care providers. They may want to be in control yet they feel compelled to yield that control. Stemming from the glut of information about the way that they can and should be with their health care providers, relational paradoxes abound for patients. Frankel (1984) suggested that "as members of a culture, physicians and patients are . . . faced with the practical interactional task of demonstrating that knowledge appropriately *in* the world" (p. 136). If there is no one way to be a competent patient, how can patients present themselves as "competent"?

Health caregivers deal with such irreconcilable paradoxes as well. Although they are no longer overtly indoctrinated by the traditional medical model in medical school, caregivers still must take some degree of charge of the interview in order to complete examinations, to gain the patient history, and importantly, to offer recommendations. However, the paradox lies in their dual commitment to trying to treat the patient and trying to empower the patient to take responsibility and to make personal choices. If the doctor believes that preventative screenings are important or that surgery is needed, how does that doctor balance the need for lobbying for that course of action with the desire to let the patient take ownership of the ultimate decision, especially when patients and their relatives seem so ready to engage in litigation if anything goes wrong? Although we know enough to recognize that the static role of doctor as compliance-gainer is inadequate, the wealth of information and possibilities for interactional choices sparks ambiguity and paradox, not the safety net of a rigid role with set goals.

Individuals in the postmodern era find themselves in perhaps the ultimate Pandora's box, fragmented by the potentiality of identities and realities, no longer able to accept singularity of self-definition, no longer able to clearly define "right" from "wrong," "black" from "white." The purity of absolutism has shifted to the shadows of ambiguity. A loss of commitment to objectivity and singularity of positions and selves is implicit to living in the postmodern era (see Gergen, 1991; Seidman, 1994).

The advent of postmodernism makes relational communication even more important yet difficult for interactional partners, especially in an institutionalized context such as health care encounters. In contrast to previous conceptions of health care encounters, institutional roles exist only as interactants co-create and perpetuate them during interactions. As caregivers and patients interact during health care encounters, they necessarily rely on the reflexivity of language (not institutional mandates or static relational definitions) to achieve co-orientation to their roles as health care interactants. In so doing, they engage in the temporal process of indicating their intersubjective, temporal understanding of "what is going on here," "who are we to each other," and "how do we legitimately treat each other in this situation at this particular fraction of time."

Stemming from their taken-for-granted assumption of what constitutes each role (see Garfinkel, 1967; Goffman, 1959), caregivers and patients behave, verbally and nonverbally, and simultaneously offer definitions of the nature of the medical encounter and their roles within that encounter. As Heritage (1984) suggested, "It is via the reflexive properties of actions that the participants . . . find themselves in a world whose characteristics they are visibly and describably engaged in producing and reproducing. . . ." (p. 110).

Because participants attempt to make their actions consistent with what they envision a doctor or patient would do, caregivers and patients utilize conversational resources to make their behaviors accountable as instances of "being a patient" or "being a doctor" (see Frankel, 1990; Garfinkel, 1967; Heritage, 1984; Zimmerman & Pollner, 1970). As Garfinkel (1967) clarified, "By his accounting practices the member makes familiar, commonplace activities of everyday life recognizable *as* familiar, commonplace activities . . ." (pp. 9–10).

However, efforts to make something accountable as "legitimate" role behavior necessarily fall short of complete because of the fragmentation of the postmodern era; thus, interactants must continually re-interpret what constitutes "acceptable," "permittable," and "viable" enactments of any given preferred role, while also dealing with the jumbled nature of their scattered selves that precludes singularity of self (for related writings on the situated accomplishment of individual and relational identities, see Beck, 1995; Goffman, 1959; Katovich, 1986; Tracy & Carjuzaa, 1993; Tracy & Naughton, 1994; Wieder & Pratt, 1990). The institution and institutional roles may no longer be taken for granted in terms of "correct," pre-defined situational, relational, or role definitions; instead, they must be treated as active, ongoing co-

constructions by the participants—participants who also come to the encounter as constantly emerging entities without static, singular self-definitions (see Fisher & Groce, 1990; Shotter & Gergen, 1994).

By taking a postmodern perspective of relational communication in health care encounters, we build on Bateson's application of systems theory to communication. In particular, we embrace the idea of caregiver–patient relationships as emergent, processual, interdependent, and consequential; we pursue the "pattern(s) which connect" (see Bateson, 1951, 1979) the interactants and facilitate the system. However, we do so while recognizing the potential of paradox and ambiguity in terms of the multiplicity of relational roles and definitions, in terms of fluid system boundaries, and in terms of diverse goals. In so doing, we go beyond Mishler's (1984) description of "dialectical tensions" between social and medical lifeworlds. Although Baxter and Montgomery (1996) provide a bridge from the traditional conception of dialectical tension as binary opposites to a more complex dynamic, we contend that viewing identities as tensions still harkens back to a more modernist construct, still implying separateness (as opposed to concurrence) of identities, goals, and preferences. Interactants struggle with the both–and-ness of the postmodern condition; fragments of their individual and relational identities may clash, but they cannot shift from one identity and abandon the other one, hence the potential paradox *with* (not tension *between*) identities.

Thus, interactants work to co-create more than just "a" system with set roles, rules, and boundaries; in the fog of a multiplicity of possibilities, they must somehow co-determine what dimensions of their mutual relationship as well as what aspects of their lives and goals may emerge as relevant at any given time. For example, the patient is not either a patient *or* a woman *or* a family member *or* a professional *or* a consumer; the essence of that woman encompasses *all* of those pieces of her life in addition to the diverse goals and attitudes and desires that accompany and extend beyond those roles.

Given the multiplicity of possible preferred relational and individual identities and goals, the challenge for health care interactants is to collaboratively co-construct a relational dynamic that enables them to manage the fragments of those identities and goals that they mutually desire to come forth and to be addressed during any given encounter. Importantly, like viewing a kaleidoscope, interactants cannot bring all of the fragments of their individual and relational identities into focus at once; the fragments blur, overlap, and meld together too much. However, also like a kaleidoscope, those dimensions of interactants' individual and relational identities do not disappear when not in focus but instead remain lurking just beneath the surface.

A perpetual close-up on one aspect of their possible selves and their relationship limits the potential for paradox, but it hinders a more comprehensive understanding of who they are and what they want from the interaction and from each other. Both frustration with the traditional medical model and discontent with efforts to shift from that model to a more holistic one stem from such a singularity in focus.

The very modernist traditional medical model, which emphasizes a quite narrow view of the doctor–patient relationship, denies both practitioners and their patients who accept that model the opportunity to treat each other beyond their strict medical roles (see Federman, 1990; Kallen & Stephenson, 1981; Korsch, Gozzi, & Negrete, 1968). For example, as the story earlier in this chapter indicated, Amanda entered the hospital for treatment. The examination that she received may well have facilitated subsequent treatment. In fact, doctors who adhere to the traditional medical model may view the examination as appropriate; the doctors gained the information that they needed to ascertain the patient's problem. Amanda did not attempt to introduce alternative perspectives of what should transpire. Stunned by their approach, she stayed silent. Furthermore, her silence may have been responsive to cultural conditioning (as well as to the relational positioning that these doctors did through their nonverbal and lack of verbal interaction with Amanda) that doctors are authority figures who can do as they want and who should not be challenged. If she had reacted differently (i.e., by asking questions or even by disconfirming the manner in which she was being treated by the doctors), the challenge to their monolithic view of her and the encounter may very well have prompted a response by the doctors that was similar to that of one doctor who examined me.

I had selected a high-risk pregnancy specialist for my care during my fourth pregnancy. After two miscarriages, I was determined that I would leave little to chance. During this particular visit, I was still in the "danger zone" of the first trimester, and I was highly nervous about the status of the pregnancy and my odds for carrying this baby to term. Unfortunately, my regular doctor was at a conference so one of his colleagues at the high-risk clinic was assigned to visit with his patients during this time.

I did not have the opportunity to meet the doctor before our visit, but I had been greatly impressed by the overall professionalism of the staff at this clinic. The technology was state-of-the-art; the nurses were efficient, and my regular doctor had been wonderfully reassuring about the potential success of this pregnancy. I felt as though I was in the best hands possible, and yet I wanted continual information about how this baby was doing, and, especially given the experience that I described in Chapter 1, I needed to feel involved and participative in the decisions about my baby's care. I knew that this clinic had contributed to the birth of a great number of "miracle babies," but selfishly, I cared only about my miracle baby at that time.

I did not have long to wait before the substitute doctor charged through the door. He brushed by me as I sat on the examining table, wearing only a sheer hospital gown. He never looked me. If he had, he would have seen a petite woman with a youthful face. If he had looked still deeper, he would have noticed the fear in my eyes and the tense lines that crowd my face when I worry.

He put my chart down on the counter at the opposite side of the room. Flipping through the pages, he started asking me questions; however, he never let me complete my answers. "How far along are you?" he asked. "Eight weeks," I responded. "Why were you referred to us?" he asked. "Well, I went through 3 years of infertility, and they—" I started. "Well, you're pregnant now," he interrupted. I tried to explain again. "Yes, but I had two miscarriages, and we think—" I said. He interrupted again, still looking down, "Oh so we've got you on the progesterone. That working for you?" "Yes," I replied, "but when—" "Good, okay, so—" he said.

Frustrated, I cut him off this time. "Are you interested in my response," I asked. For the first time, the doctor looked at me, albeit briefly, and then said, "yes," and he paused. I started again. "I have never taken it before, and I was wondering—" "Well, we'll keep you on it for 12 weeks," he stated, again not letting me complete my request for information.

I sat up as straight as I could on the table, turned to him, and said in a style from my days in debate, "Look, I don't know who you think you're dealing with, but I'm not a stupid female; I'm not ignorant. I am a professor. I have a PhD in communication, and I study doctor–patient interactions, particularly in the women's health care context, and frankly, you suck." He turned to me quickly at that point. His face was red, and his body was rigid. Quietly, he said, "What?" I took a deep breath and hoped that he could not see my heart pounding through that skimpy little gown. "Look, this is important to me. I know enough to know that I am still not out of the woods. I need to have you listen to me. I want you to have all of the information that you need so that you can help this little baby make it. I won't take that long, but I absolutely need for you to listen to me and to tell me what I need to know." He just continued to stare at me as his face turned increasingly red.

We managed to get through the encounter without further incident but also with quite a bit of silence. At my next visit, my regular doctor smiled and told me of the substitute doctor's report that I had given him a "hard time." When I protested that depiction of the encounter, my doctor gave the account that the substitute is "just not used to dealing with patients like you." However, as I reflect on that encounter, I realize that the substitute was just not used to treating patients holistically, recognizing the complexity of individual patients which goes well beyond medical complaints. Implicitly, through the way in which he interacted with me, that doctor denied all identities and goals beyond that of a specific type of patient with a certain medical complaint. Furthermore, the doctor was likely "just not used" to having that rigid situational and relational definition challenged by his patients. My response to the doctor's constant interruptions overtly worked to indicate my preference to re-define that narrow conception of me. I argued not only that I was more than "just a patient"; I stressed that I was a person with particular needs and a consumer with specific goals.

By advocating the move from a modernist to a postmodernist conception of health care encounters, we necessarily suggest a situation in which health caregivers and their patients strive to manage interactions amidst implicit paradoxes in terms of relational definitions and perhaps in terms of goals. Even if both participants want to treat the encounter as multidimensional and to facilitate multiple goals, they inherently struggle with how they can allow aspects of their fragmented individual and relational identities to emerge, how they can display their preferences for accomplishing often diverse and contradictory goals, without disconfirming and potentially discouraging the surfacing of other bits of their relational identity.

CONSEQUENTIALITY OF RELATIONAL ACTIVITIES

In the complex context of health care encounters, then, interactants do not simply exchange content information. Even individuals who come to health care encounters with a modernist, narrow view of "the" way that the encounter should ensue still engage in verbal and nonverbal communication that suggests that particular relational definition. Through artful relational activities, interactants indicate their preferences for what aspect(s) of themselves they would like to treat as relevant in the interaction. Furthermore, through those relational activities, interactants implicitly respond to parts of the others' preferred relational and individual definitions and in so doing affirming or disconfirming them (see Watzlawick et al., 1967).

In the earlier example, both the doctor's initial treatment of me and my subsequent challenge to that treatment constituted instances of disconfirmation of at least some part of the other's preferred identity and goals for the encounter. Instead of a gentle carving of what splinters of our individual identities and our relationship should be addressed (as opposed to other possible chips of our respective and collective identities), we both axed our way into modernist absolutism. The doctor denied my attempts to participate; I questioned his authority to do so as well as his qualifications as a health care provider. We accomplished little toward building a partnership.

As a number of scholars have observed, such disconfirmation works reflexively as a means of refining system rules and role definitions (see Cissna & Sieburg, 1981; Watzlawick et al., 1967). However, such disconfirmation also results in a threat to at least part of the other's "face" or preferred identity (Brown & Levinson, 1987; Cupach & Metts, 1994; Goffman, 1959,

1967; Ting-Toomey, 1994; Tracy, 1990). Clearly, disconfirmation does not facilitate an interactional environment where both participants collabora- tively enable each other to achieve their multiple goals, to realize their preferred individual and relational identities, and most importantly, to work toward a partnership for quality health care for the woman patient.

In this book, we strive to describe how interactants may jointly co-produce an environment that is conducive for a partnership orientation while recog- nizing that the partner aspect of the relational dynamic is certainly not the only relevant relational definition or relational goal. The postmodern per- spective of relational communication that we outline in this chapter guides our exploration of how health caregivers and their patients reciprocally facilitate, or do not facilitate, fragments of their preferred individual and relational identities to emerge. We stress that it is through the interactive co-accomplishment of relational activities such as face management, iden- tification, interactional framing, humor, and so on, that the multiplicity of relational and individual identities and goals may be realized by health caregivers and their patients.

The following chapters provide descriptions of how health caregivers and their patients display and co-accomplish their respective relational, medical, and educational goals, in light of the complexity, ambiguity, and potential paradoxes of postmodern living and the multiplicity of identities. Although these goals are divided for organizational purposes in this book, we view them as very much intertwined and interdependent, and we conclude this project by detailing the reflexivity of each of these goals in terms of the other goals as well as in terms of the emergent relational and individual identities of the health care participants.

Co-Accomplishment
of Relational Goals

As part of ethnographic data collection at a hospital, I was shadowing "Linda," one of the nurses in the OB-GYN unit, when we first met "Ann," a newly admitted patient. Linda led the way through the door. She glanced around the dimly lit room, switched on one of the lights, walked to the end of the bed, and scanned Ann's chart. Ann sat on the side of the bed, legs swaying, still wearing her t-shirt and jeans.

Linda lifted her eyes from the chart, looked at Ann, and said, "Not feeling so well tonight, hmm?" Ann kept her gaze focused on the floor, and another voice answered, "No, she's not at all. She's been hurting and throwing up all day, and I just know that something's wrong." Linda looked briefly at the woman in the bedside chair who had just spoken and then shifted her gaze back to Ann.

Linda asked, "I bet that this is your mom, right, Ann?" Ann nodded. Linda continued, "Tell me how you've been feeling today, Ann. Any cramping?" Ann nodded. "Vomiting?" Ann slowly moved her head up and down, her eyes still fixed on the floor. Finally, she spoke, stating that "I just feel awful. Is it supposed to feel like this?" She paused, turned her head, peered into Linda's eyes, and, in a little girl, ever-so-quiet voice, she hesitantly asked, "Am I losing the baby?"

At the age of 13, Ann had been admitted to the hospital after coming into the emergency room and complaining of abdominal pain and vomiting. She was 4 months pregnant. Throughout Ann's exchange with Linda, Ann's mother touched Ann's leg, held her hand, and attempted to answer Linda's questions to Ann. Yet, each time that the mother offered a response instead of Ann, Linda re-directed the question to Ann.

This encounter exemplifies the complexity of relational communication during health care visits in this postmodern era. Throughout the brief 10-minute visit, Linda and Ann communicated, verbally and nonverbally, with regard to their preferences for how the encounter would ensue, for how they wanted to co-define their ever-emergent relationship, and for which fragments of their respective relational and individual identities should come forth as relevant, salient, and primary during the interaction.

For example, Ann interactionally enabled her mother and Linda to take control of the exchange. Ann mostly looked down at her feet and the floor, avoiding eye contact with Linda. She also behaved in a manner that permitted her mother to speak for her. Ann did not amend, nor add to, her mother's description of Ann's condition. Ann did not interrupt or admonish her mother as she responded to the nurse. Instead, Ann sat passively on the bed, listening to her mother talk for her and reducing her own role to offering only the most minimal of responses to Linda. In so doing, Ann facilitated her mother's participation in the encounter while not disconfirming Linda's efforts to direct what occurred and to seek information. Ann did not just sit in silence and negate Linda's implicit request for answers to her questions. She simply allowed her mother to take her turn for her. When Linda did repeat the questions even after the mother's responses, Ann did respond, albeit minimally.

Through the way in which she positioned herself during the visit, Ann indicated her preference for deference to the others in the room. She treated the situation as one in which others had the legitimate right to ask and answer questions about her. Strangely, although this entire visit was about Ann, she opted not to assume a central part, taking only a limited supporting role in this very real life drama. However, as we have noted earlier, Ann's reactions alone did not, and could not, define the multifaceted nature of the encounter. That orientation to the encounter worked in relation to Linda's and Ann's mother's contributions to the conversation to co-produce the emergent relational dynamic.

Given the nature of Ann's verbal and nonverbal behavior, Linda could have chosen to interact with Ann's mother rather than Ann. If Linda's goal was only to obtain information about Ann's condition, perhaps that would have been sufficient, and certainly more efficient, given Ann's reticence in responding. However, Linda interactionally designated Ann as the one who needed to participate. Linda marked Ann's mother's answers as lacking by refusing to accept the mother's voice as Ann's. Linda did not overtly tell the mother that Ann should speak for herself, yet Linda indicated that preference by letting the mother finish and then by posing essentially the same questions once more to Ann, repeatedly inviting Ann to talk about her condition, to take ownership of her health care concerns. Linda's recurrent questions worked both to direct the interaction as well as to demonstrate her desire for Ann to participate more actively in the encounter.

An analysis of this interaction from a traditional relational communication perspective would easily suggest that the three interactants (Ann, Ann's mother, and Linda) co-created a relational dynamic in which a primarily complementary relational pattern ensued. Linda asked questions; someone answered. Linda picked the relevant topics; others responded. Implicitly, the emergent rules of this system permitted Linda to take control and to determine the acceptability and adequacy of answers. Neither Ann nor Ann's mother ever disputed how Linda approached the encounter or the nature of her communication with them. Even after Ann's mother gave information and Linda re-directed questions again to Ann, they did not look at Linda and indignantly react with something to the effect of "asked and answered already." Linda asserted; others accepted; hence, the co-construction of a complementary relational dynamic.

However, by bringing a postmodern perspective to relational communication in health care encounters, we begin to obtain a broader picture of the daedal, reflexive nature of relational communication in this context beyond a focus on relational control. By simply noting who seems to take control and who seems to defer control to someone else, we gain only a limited depiction of the interactants as just one way or another. A postmodern perspective permits an otherwise unattainable appreciation of the complexity, multiplicity, and paradox of relational and individual identities.

For instance, after we left the room, Linda explained to me that she could not just allow Ann to depend on her mother to answer for her. Although Linda acknowledged that Ann was only 13, barely more than a child herself, Linda contended that she could not "baby" Ann. In 5 short months, Ann was going to be a mother herself, and, Linda reasoned, Ann needed to take responsibility, to understand her health situation, and to participate in health care discussions and decisions on behalf of her unborn baby. Paradoxically, Linda felt compelled to attend to her patient in terms of Ann's simultaneous yet contradictory identities as "child" as well as "woman," "daughter" as well as "prospective mom," "patient" with health concerns as well as "teen" with nonmedical fears, desires, questions, and relationships—all indistinguishably melded together, interwoven, and inseparable.

Neither Linda or Ann could totally address one identity in isolation from the others. The composite of their complicated relationship consisted of—yet also extended beyond—the potentiality of their multiple relational and individual definitions and identities. All fragments of identity impacted—and were influenced by—the others; all constrained yet facilitated the carving of who they were together at that given time. The ongoing challenge for caregivers and patients in general is to respond to the pieces of identity that surface without threatening or disconfirming the ones that lurk just beneath those that peek above (e.g., in this case, recognizing the "child" without patronizing the "almost-but-not-really" adult while treating the "prospective mom" without failing to also acknowledge the "little girl"). All fragments cannot be clearly at the surface, but the blur on the boundaries exists nonetheless.

Linda entered the examining room with her own diverse and conflicting preconceptions about the world, how people should behave, what people should do or not do. In addition, she brought assorted ideas and experiences that lent themselves to her ability to assess symptoms, derive hypotheses about medical diagnoses and possible treatments, and perform the tasks that she perceives as part of her job. That multifaceted, perhaps diverse exposure to medical knowledge also contributed to Linda's own understanding about how medical encounters should ensue and how she and the patient should treat each other.

For example, despite—and in light of—these a priori assumptions, Linda asked questions, nodded her head and took notes, affirming Ann's—and Ann's mother's—view of her situation and her condition throughout her visit with Ann. In so doing, Linda treated Ann's description of her symptoms as sincere and significant, not as an "over-reaction" or as unimportant. However, Linda told me as we were walking down the hallway from Ann's room that she did not think that Ann's pregnancy was in trouble. According to Linda, Ann likely felt discomfort because her body was young, too immature for a pregnancy yet forced to deal with one anyway. Even so, Ann would possibly carry the baby to term, despite the discomfort from which she suffered on this particular evening.

To hear Linda's perspective on Ann and her mother as we continued our journey to the nurses' station was fascinating, especially given my observation of her conversation with them. Linda spoke of her experience with other girls like Ann and their mothers during her years at this hospital, "babies" who were having babies and the mothers—would-be grandmothers—who sometimes encouraged them to do so. Linda reflected, "She's far too young to have a baby. The changes in her body are so enormous that she's not going to know what's normal to feel. No wonder she's in here tonight." Linda paused for a moment, looking around at the walls of the hospital corridor that were decorated in soft pastels. "Some want a doll to love; some just want someone to love them. Others, like that one, have a mother who wants that baby for her own reason, lots of times around here [they do so] to up the welfare check," Linda said reflectively. She stopped for a moment and then added "It's hard, you know. You can't make judgments and yet . . ." Her voice trailed off, the sentence unfinished.

We cannot know what Ann was thinking that evening as she talked with Linda. We cannot know the circumstances that led up to her trip to the hospital emergency room; we cannot know the relational or family pressures that she faced nor the nature of her relationships with others outside of that sterile hospital room. Like Linda, we only have available to us what Ann chose to reveal and how she chose to react to Linda and to her mother during our presence in the room.

However, as Linda and I went back to the nurses' station, I was struck by what Linda opted to make relevant during her talk with Ann. An employee of a Catholic hospital, a well-educated woman, an experienced nurse in an economically disadvantaged region of the country, an individual with a potpouri of political convictions and social perspectives, Linda did not scold, preach, or chastise. She did not comment on Ann's morality or economic status or choices in a society where unprotected premarital sex can lead to consequences far more disastrous than an unexpected—perhaps unwanted—pregnancy.

Some may argue that Linda was "just being professional." We agree that she behaved in a manner that could be construed as professional; however, Linda cannot be narrowly defined only in terms of her job as a health caregiver, nor according to some preconceived view about what behaviors constitute "professional." We think that it is ironic, given the current emphasis on holism in medicine, that the pervasive tendency by patients and scholars is to treat caregivers monolithically, restricting them to only a medical role and denying the array of goals, emotions, perspectives, and identities that expand beyond—yet still include—their occupational position as caregivers. Such a narrow casting of caregivers inherently limits an understanding of how caregivers may respond and what they must struggle with during encounters.

Despite that limitation, however, it makes sense for both caregivers and patients to embrace singular, static conceptions rather than confront ambiguity. Although simultaneously desiring a caring, compassionate person who can reach out to them and to understand them, patients may well prefer the "expert" over the fallible human being, the tunnel-visioned professional to the fragmented individual. (In fact, caregivers may feel more confident and secure by presenting themselves as a focused authority.) By taking an either–or stance—as opposed to a both–and one—patients, caregivers, and scholars avoid paradoxes that emerge from trying to view these seemingly incompatible, incongruent sets of opposites as reconcilable and co-existing (i.e., both expert and fallible, both tunnel-visioned and fragmented). They do so, however, at the expense of a more complete appreciation of the complex person who happens to wear a stethoscope. Hence, the conundrum of rejecting the traditional medical model—patients want caregivers to treat them holistically yet, for patients to view caregivers in a like manner, they open up the possibility that caregivers may not have all of the answers; they may be flawed people as well.

Although we want caregivers to be professional, we doubt that either patients or scholars or caregivers really want caregivers to be confined to only that isolated fragment of their selves (as if that was possible anyway).

If we really could command caregivers to turn off the other aspects of themselves at will like a water faucet (a task that none of us may accomplish in this era of perpetual and confusing overlap), most of us would leave health care encounters thirsting for richer experiences than question-and-answer sessions.

This is not to say that some—perhaps still many—caregivers focus strictly on medical tasks during interactions with their patients, silencing overt references to other aspects of themselves even though those other dimensions subtly flavor the manner in which medical tasks get done. The belief that monolithic self-presentations—and singularity of representation—of caregivers and patients are possible has been the outcome of the traditional medical model. However, we believe that setting up the rigid dialectic of depicting those who offer care as "professionals" or "regular people" is as much of a false dichotomy as treating those who seek care as either "patients" or "regular people," with as significant of consequences for the interaction during health care encounters. We contend that caregivers, like their patients, should be appreciated as multidimensional and that caregivers come to encounters as *both* professionals *and* as individuals who have experienced life, relationships, and information beyond medical texts. It is because identities may not be isolated, but rather link together—albeit incongruently, that the same mix of experiences in their lives that would enable caregivers to understand patients, to identity with patients, to work with patients as partners on some level may also prove to be paradoxical for caregivers as they strive to do so.

In this case, amidst Linda's own diverse perspectives, mixed feelings, and multiplicity of individual identities, her interactional choices worked to cocreate with Ann a relational dynamic in which Ann was a participant and in which Linda was a facilitator, not a preacher nor a judge. From what Linda knew about Ann, and in light of her own conflicting opinions about Ann and her pregnancy, Linda undertook the task of interactionally working to empower Ann to participate as an adult while also caring for and not disconfirming the scared little girl who found herself in a new, very grown-up situation.

Yet, Linda faced the difficulty of interacting with Ann as a complex individual without really gaining much insight into Ann as a multidimensional person. Importantly, even though not all possible relational and individual identities come into focus during health care encounters, they certainly do not disappear for the participants. Because individuals do not shift among (but instead encompass all) fragments of identities in their chaotic lives, their interactional partners must participate in a virtual haze—not knowing all aspects of the other's scattered life yet walking through a foggy minefield where missteps could prove face-threatening or hurtful for some unknown dimension of that other.

PARADOXICAL NATURE OF RELATIONAL GOALS

The forenoted example of a health care encounter reinforces four key arguments from Chapter 2. First, in this postmodern era, interactants come together for brief instances, torn and confused by the chaos of a plethora of possible identities. However, those identities do not consist of static, pre-set roles that are rigid and distinct. Because of the over-abundance of available—yet contradictory—information and influence, identities are fluid, fragmented, emergent, and multifaceted. Without a consistency of what constitutes "right" and "wrong," "good" or "bad" self-presentations that fit a preferred identity (e.g., what verbal or nonverbal behaviors are those of a "good" doctor, a "good" patient), interactants face the ongoing struggle of working collaboratively to co-construct who they are, and perhaps more importantly, who they are to each other at any given place and time, in any given situation.

Borrowing from Gadamer's (1975, 1976, 1988) writings on hermeneutics, we believe that interactants continually engage in re-interpretations of their perpetually unsettled relationships and identities; they cannot label them in particular ways and assume that their meanings never change. Instead, as interactants continually and temporally re-experience each other and themselves, they essentially and necessarily re-interpret "what is going on here," "who are we," and "who are we to each other."

Second, those emergent, co-created relational identities (i.e., the co-definition(s) of the relationship between the participants—who they are to each other) and the also emergent, co-created individual identities (i.e., the co-definition(s) of each individual interactant) are inherently intertwined. As did Bateson (1951), we approach relational communication as systemic; each of the participants is interrelated with the other participants, and the relationship is something that is substantially different from, and greater than, the sum of each of the individual participants—the concept of nonsummativity. As such, the ways in which the participants co-define the relationship also impact and constrain the nature of individual identities within that relationship at that given time—although, paradoxically in our postmodern view of relational communication, those participants never lose any bits of their individual identities.

For example, the focus at a particular moment in a caregiver–patient interaction may be on the caregiver's identity as an expert and the patient's identity as a consumer; the emergent relational definition at that moment in time highlights that particular dimension of their relationship. The relational and individual identities are inseparable and interdependent. However, whereas those identities shift to the surface, their respective other identities also co-exist. Because fragments of identity are so tangled together, those other identities likely even flavor how each creatively constructs her self-presentation as "expert" and "consumer" and how each responds to the other as they collaboratively achieve consensus on a dimension of their relationship.

It is because roles are not statically set and because of the complexity and multiplicity of identities that, third, we can only rely on what individuals make available to their interactional partners with regard to their preferences for how they want to be treated and to treat others and for how they want the encounter to ensue. Because interactants cannot possibly make relevant every dimension of their lives at once, they display, through their verbal and nonverbal behaviors and the nature of their reactions to other participants, what dimensions of their lives are especially salient at any given moment. As the interactants do so, they also work to co-create what aspects of their relationship should come into focus at that point in time. Our concentration on interaction in the following pages is quite consistent with what everyday interactants have available to them (and importantly, do not have accessible to them) as they converse with others. For interactants, the rub lies not so much in responding to what others say and do and continually working toward shared meaning of a multitude of activities; it stems from what they fail to learn, what does not initially emerge as relevant at a time but which, because it still just drifts on the periphery, can be a wound to be opened, not-too-old scars to be pricked like a thorn.

The conversation that I had with the obstetrician who was substituting for my regular doctor constitutes a good exemplar. That doctor certainly should have let me answer his questions completely without interruption, regardless of my plethora of professional, personal, educational, or medical experiences. However, because he did not sit down, talk with me, discover my needs and concerns, and make an effort to grasp the complicated person within the body (and because he did not give me a lot of opportunity to volunteer such information), his questions zipped toward me like bullets. Implicitly, he had threatened my preferred identities—a responsible consumer, caring mom, good patient, knowledgeable professional, educated woman, and viable partner.

I was ambushed by his disconfirming demeanor, wanting to put up my defenses, desiring to re-define the situation, myself, and my relational dynamic with the doctor. Even more so, I felt re-injured from previous indignities in health care encounters and from my own frustration with not contributing more during those health care situations. The agonizing hurt and painful feelings of loss and helplessness flooded through my mind, and my defenses shot straight up. I was not going to be victimized nor was I going to behave like a victim. I fought back by overtly challenging his treatment and his definition of me, the situation, and our relational dynamic. By not responding to me as a multidimensional person and by not discovering the depth of my prior experiences beyond technical, medical descriptions on my chart, he unknowingly jabbed a part of me that, despite its salience in my life, did not leap to the surface again during the pregnancy. Given that his speciality is in high-risk pregnancies, I wonder how many other women have visited with this doctor and choked back anger as he trampled bits of their selves that he did not bother to discover nor attempt to accommodate.

It is precisely because of the ambiguity, the uncertainty, the complexity, the confusion, the fragmentation, and the multiplicity of identities and relationships in this postmodern era that, fourth, interactants must inherently deal with paradoxes of relational and individual identities. The both–and-ness of those identities forces a situation where interactants highlight aspects that are relevant but where a profusion of other identities skulk just out of direct view, hidden in the shadows but waiting to appear.

The paradox of relational identities stems from contradictions among identities. Individuals' fragmented selves may encompass identities that seem incompatible, but, because individuals cannot be one or another but rather both simultaneously, individuals—like their interactional partners—must continuously reckon with the inconsistency. For example, how can caregivers and patients co-accomplish a relationship that accommodates both a relational definition that stems from the differential in expertise (and thus, the caregiver's "right" to direct the interaction, to obtain more personal information than she or he likely gives to the patient, to recommend a plan of action, etc.) as well as a relational definition that stems from an appreciation of similarity in other experiences—like woman–woman, neighbor–neighbor, community member–community member, colleague–colleague (and thus, where both contribute equally to the direction and nature of the conversation)? How can caregivers and patients collaboratively nurture a relationship that accommodates a relational definition wherein both interactants work as partners amidst the concurrent desire to treat each other in ways that come from a diverse number of influences (i.e., a patient's preference to show deference to the caregiver's "authority" while asserting her own views, perspectives, and goals)?

THE REFLEXIVITY OF RELATIONAL ACTIVITIES

As we detail in this chapter, caregivers and patients struggle with three simultaneous, yet reflexive and interdependent sets of relational accomplishments during health care encounters. Caregivers and patients co-accomplish *relational definitions* (such as a partner–partner dynamic) through various *relational activities*. Those relational activities (such as facework, identification, and interactional framing) are co-achieved by the interactants through *conversational activities* (such as affirmation of a multiplicity of patient identities—via verbal recognition of patient opinions, humorous acknowledgment of paradoxes of identity for the patient, and nonmedical task talk and allusions to commonalities—as well as a multiplicity of caregiver identities—via personal disclosures and directives). In this chapter, we provide exemplars of all but the nature of directives, which we discuss in Chapter 4 on patient education.

Through this co-accomplishment of individual identities, the interactants inherently engage in the process of positioning and re-positioning themselves relationally; one set of identities cannot be enacted without relational and systemic consequences for the other co-interactants. Furthermore, although we highlight these conversational activities as "relational activities" here, we stress that the interactional work toward (and co-orientation that gets displayed through) the attainment of educational and medical goals also reflexively shape relational definitions. Although, by organizational necessity, we speak of these identities, goals, and activities—both relational and conversational—separately, we stress that they are much like an intricate web, not a smooth circle where, for example, one set of activities simply and linearly connects to another. Instead, we suggest that they are intertwined, interdependent, and reflexive; again, borrowing from Watzlawick et al. (1967), we view every attribute of and contribution to the emergent dynamic between the interactants as important, salient, and consequential.

In this chapter, we take a micro-analytic approach to understanding how caregivers and patients can co-construct an interactional environment that facilitates a partnership-like aspect of the ever-fluid relational dynamic. We begin by describing the importance of these relational activities (facework, identification, and interactional framing) for the attainment of particular, preferred relational and individual identities and goals, given the complexity of interpersonal relationships in this postmodern era. We then offer exemplars of how caregivers and patients in our data sets co-produce or not produce conversational activities that enable them to realize or not realize relational activities (and subsequently, relational definitions).

Facework

In his dramaturgical perspective of social interaction, Erving Goffman (1955, 1959, 1967, 1972) described the efforts of social actors to be taken and treated in particular ways by their interactional counterparts. Goffman (1955, 1959) suggested that individuals advance a certain social *face* by behaving in a manner that can legitimately be taken by others in their culture as a special type of person. Individuals may do so by dressing one way (as opposed to other ways), by affiliating with distinct others (and marking that affiliation in artful ways that are consistent with how individuals in that collection of people display association with each other), by speaking and acting in a certain manner, or by taking part in some events—as opposed to other ones (see Goffman, 1955, 1959, 1967). Through their own specialized understanding of role enactment, individuals advance their preferred social face.

However, as Goffman (1955, 1959, 1967) and others (Brown & Levinson, 1987; Craig, Tracy, & Spisak, 1986; Cupach & Metts, 1994; Ting-Toomey, 1994; Tracy, 1990) argued, face is an interactional, not an individual, construct. Goffman (1955, 1967) maintained that interactants display how they want to be taken and that others must respond to that self-positioning. Most of the research on facework and politeness has concentrated on the care that social actors tend to have for the face of others—although acknowledging the efforts that individuals make to try to abstain from situations or behaviors that could prove to be embarrassing. Brown and Levinson (1987) explained that interactants engage in a *cost-benefit* analysis of potentially threatening the face of another individual wherein the cost of somehow calling the individual's face into question must be less than the price of not doing so at all. Although Brown and Levinson's (1987) model of politeness has received some criticism with regard to validity issues (see Tracy & Baratz, 1994), their theory of politeness has served as a catalyst for research on how "politeness" gets accomplished and how "embarrassment" gets deterred, mostly in terms of "strategies" for politeness (see Aronsson & Satterlund-Larsson, 1987; Baxter, 1984; Cupach & Metts, 1994; Edelmann, 1994; Satterlund-Larsson, Johanson, & Svardsudd, 1994; Shimanoff, 1988, 1994, as well as discussions by Lim, 1994, and Ting-Toomey & Cocroft, 1994). In fact, Goffman (1955, 1967) contended that facework permeates everyday conversation as individuals strive to help others to avoid embarrassment and to realize their preferred face:

> Just as the member of any group is expected to have self-respect, so also he is expected to sustain a standard of considerateness. . . . This kind of mutual acceptance seems to be a basic structural feature of interaction, especially the interaction of face-to-face talk. (Goffman, 1955, pp. 215–216)

However, this focus on how individuals support or threaten the face of others has been at the expense of a more complete appreciation of the ramifications of face for the constantly evolving relational identities of the dyad. Despite this, the conceptualization of face as reciprocally co-defined that has been prevalent in the facework/politeness literature fits well with the writings by Bateson and the Palo Alto Group that were described in Chapter 2. If the dyad can be considered a system, and if the interactants within that system position themselves in relation to each other, then the interactional work of one individual in the dyad forces a response—an affirmation or disconfirmation of how that individual is promoting him or herself and, thus simultaneously and reflexively, how that individual is treating the relationship and his or her relational partner. That response is consequential to the second partner's face and to the accomplishment of an intersubjective relational definition.

In the case of health care encounters, for example, if one interactant (likely the caregiver) presents him or herself as "the expert," then the possible interactional and relational choices for the other interactant (likely the patient) are necessarily minimized if that second interactant opts not to challenge or dispute the first interactant's self presentation. Hence, because of the relational nature of face, the affirmation or disconfirmation of another's preferred face—a face that becomes discernable through his or her verbal and nonverbal behaviors, choice of activities, dress, associations, and so on—impacts, constrains, and works reflexively to define the dyadic system as well as the face of the affirmer or disconfirmer (for related argument, see Watzlawick et al., 1967).

For example, Goffman (1955, 1967) described how acts of deference work to reify the position of individuals in relation to each other. He also noted how "corrections" for failure to demonstrate "appropriate" deference—while face-threatening to the one who "failed"—reinforce the preferred face of the corrector (who exercises the "right" to correct the other, thus challenging the face of that other). The relational implicativeness of face and facework underlies the co-construction of the relational dynamic (i.e., who the participants are to each other, what may and may not be legitimately said or done to the other, etc.).

In addition to the scant scholarship on ramifications of face and facework for the dyad in face and politeness literature, a troubling trend has been to ignore the multidimensional nature of individuals and relationships in this body of work. Although Penman (1994) referred briefly to postmodernism in her writing on face, she constituted a notable exception. As discussed earlier in this chapter and in Chapter 2, monolithic treatments of face (i.e., casting face as singular in terms of potentiality) avoid recognizing the complexity of living and interacting in this postmodern era as well as the multiplicity of possible identities, thus oversimplifying the abundance of choices and issues for contemporary interactants. Hence, in our work here, we use previous research and theoretical arguments on face and facework as a point of departure for our own postmodern view of the relational and individual identities that emerge during health care encounters.

We take the position that the idea of "facework" is important in—in fact, vital to—understanding interactions in the women's health care context; however, we maintain that the interactional means through which caregivers and their patients display and co-achieve preferred identities (as well as politeness and other-directed facework) function reflexively to impact multiple identities, not simply *an* identity, *a* relational definition. Thus, our goal here is to examine the aspects of facework that can contribute to a multiplicity of individual identities and a multiplicity of relational identities, not singularity in terms of either individuals or their emergent relationships.

Especially in the women's health care context, the potential for face threats is high, and the price of such threats can be enormous (see Alexander & McCullough, 1981; Domar, 1985–1986; Emerson, 1970; Fang, Hillard, Lindsay, & Underwood, 1984; Leserman & Luke, 1982; Ragan, 1990; Ragan & Glenn, 1990; Summey & Hurst, 1986; Weiss & Meadow, 1979). If fragments of preferred individual and relational identities are either overtly disconfirmed or subtly disregarded, then embarrassment, frustration, disappointment, and perhaps, even mistrust and anger can taint the relational dynamic between caregivers and patients and can hinder the co-accomplishment of the multiplicity of relational, educational and medical goals that both bring to their health care interactions.

Yet, the very nature of health care interactions poses inherent face risks. Consider the typical health care encounter: The patient sits in the examining room—often forced to wait for the caregiver to arrive. When the caregiver does walk into the room, the patient likely experiences a first meeting with that person (see Arntson, 1989). The advent of joint practices and community-based health care clinics hinder the ability of patients to visit with the same caregiver each time, even if they return to the same facility; the trend toward specialization rather than general practice also obstructs continuity, and holism of care by one caregiver. Like the rest of their lives, the way in which patients tend to seek and to obtain health care is scattered and sporadic.

Thus, as the patient and doctor greet each other, they must engage in specific and necessary medical business, starting with the need for the doctor to ask and for the patient to explain the reason for the visit (see comprehensive review and analysis of the first few moments of doctor–patient interactions by Modaff, 1995). The entire orientation of this time of information-giving is predominantly asymmetrical and, to use Bateson's term, "complementary"; caregivers inquire, and patients respond.

Profound asymmetry is problematic in terms of the emergence of a possible partnership dimension in the caregiver–patient relationship for a number of relational reasons. Yet, the asymmetry with regard to self-disclosure becomes particularly difficult in light of the general dispreference for differentials in self-disclosure between interactional partners, especially during initial interactions. Despite the general tendency not to self-disclose or to do so tentatively during initial encounters, patients must reveal intimate details of their private lives to caregivers—usually without reciprocation. Given the ambiguity of postmodern relationships, both interactants likely experience uncertainty about each other, about expectations, and about preconceptions, and the temporality and complexity of contemporary relationships belies efforts to learn "everything" and to eliminate apprehension about gaps. Yet, when caregivers get information and patients do not, another aspect of the knowledge differential gets reified and perpetuated, and in so doing, the interactants display part of their orientation to the relational dynamic and to their respective co-achievement of individual identities.

Compelled by the caregiver and the medical aspect of the situation, the patient does disclose. After all, the caregiver requires information in order to proceed with the offering of care. However, paradoxically, the initial meeting aspect of the situation may make disclosures seem awkward and imbalanced, thus potentially threatening fragments of the patient's identities as she strives—but may be unable—to present herself in preferred ways. As she discloses to someone who does not, the patient finds herself in the dark, struggling to stumble on to the path to more clarity; the patient may have little idea how her utterances are being construed by the caregiver nor what the caregiver wants or expects from her. However, she passes by lanterns that could afford her some sort of illumination on the interaction. Similar to many patients, she could perceive asking questions to gain information or to grasp some glimmer of the caregiver's perspective as more hazardous to aspects of her self than falling over something that she does not see in the darkness. In everyday life, interactants tend to reciprocate with regard to level of self-disclosure, and thus, patients may want the sharing and disclosing process in health care interactions to include such reciprocity. Yet, the "caregiver asks–patient answers" model often results in caregivers disclosing much less than patients. To continue to self-disclose to the caregiver while feeling uncomfortable about doing so (because of her diverse albeit simultaneous views on the need and appropriateness of self-disclosure), the patient may struggle with mixed feelings and, perhaps, embarrassment about the nature of her disclosures.

The discommodious tension is magnified by the reality that, in any health care encounter that necessitates some degree of disrobing, women patients may certainly feel vulnerable and anxious (see Goffman's work on personal "territory," 1967, 1972). In many circumstances, their bodies are covered only by a sheer piece of cloth as they talk in rooms with strangers—or at best, people with whom they have had only minimal contact. Even if the examination is only one that requires the doctor to see and touch the back or the chest or the stomach, the patient is nonetheless permitting touch in areas that most people do not get to simply feel at a first meeting; it is, as Goffman (1972) explains, a matter of personal territory. Especially for women, who have been socialized to guard themselves and their dignity and privacy, the territory issue is very salient during health care encounters in general.

Because of the way that the patient might normally limit touch and contact within the immediate area around her body when she interacts with others in everyday life, she might feel apprehensive about making so much of herself visually and physically available to the caregiver. After all, her body is her own; it constitutes a sacred area that no one has the right to invade. However, paradoxically, simultaneously, she also likely believes that the medical context in general makes such disclosure—both in terms of information and physical accessibility—legitimate and necessary.

Thus, the patient battles the both–and-ness of space without truly being able to feel completely comfortable with the compromise of in-between-ness, not absolutism, in terms of *her* space yet *shared* space and in terms of the only partial possible realization of preferred identities in such a scenario. To some extent, she must willingly, albeit unwillingly, permit this stranger to come into her territory, her private space that includes her body as well as the personal distance that surrounds it. Especially during gynecologic examinations, that infringement is even more intense and potentially disconcerning (see Billings & Stoeckle, 1977; Emerson, 1970; Livingston & Ostrow, 1978; Smilkstein, DeWolfe, Erwin, McIntyre, & Shuford, 1980; for related work, see Satterlund-Larsson, Johanson, & Svardsudd, 1994). As Ragan (1990) observed, "The goal of face-protecting is particularly felt in a procedure which possibly is seen by both interactants as invasive, intruding on one's personal space and privacy, and culturally taboo" (p. 70).

The fact that she must yield her guard of her territory in the examining room contributes to a reinforcement of, as well as a concurrent potential threat to, the patient's multiplicity of identities, especially those that value control and equality. In the examining room, defenses may be diminished because of the medical necessity of disregarding personal space. Yet, paradoxically, it still *does* disconfirm that space, and it happens within the perimeters of another person's area—the caregiver's.

The examining room functions as the caregiver's own territory. The caregiver easily accesses equipment, paper supplies, and so on, directs other health care professionals, and decides where and when participants move around the room. It is within that physical area that the caregiver accomplishes his or her job and works to advance and achieve his or her own collection of individual and relational identities. In light of cultural expectations and pervasive interactional treatments of that space, the examining room has been historically considered and responded to as the caregiver's "home court." In the movie *The American President*, the President refers to the White House as the ultimate "home court advantage." We would argue that the intimidating nature of the doctor's office—the caregiver moving with ease amidst the plethora of equipment that is foreign to the patient, the patient viewing as a spectator on top of uncomfortable furniture—constitutes a similar "home court advantage." This situation promotes an inherently face-threatening situation for patients who yearn for the chance to be taken as an active participant.

However, we must stress again that even issues like personal territory should not be shoved aside as simple, singular, or statically defined. Certainly, the patient's body is her domain; the room is the caregiver's turf, and yet, the patient and caregiver confront the paradox of sharing each territory during the encounter although also preserving their respective orientations to each area as individual as well. Just as in (and actually, as part of) their relational system, the interactants must continually, interactionally, co-define how they will mutually treat these territories while juggling the ambiguity and paradox of both–and-ness—they are both individual and common space simultaneously during the encounter. Yet, the difficulty in managing these co-realities yields fertile ground for face issues because of the implicativeness and reflexivity of treatments of territory for individual and relational identities.

The tension about discrepancies in level of self-disclosure and management of personal and mutual space combine with other factors that contribute to face needs and wants. The patient might be stressed about her medical situation, uncertain about what to do or what to expect (in terms of possible medical diagnoses, treatment recommendations and relationship with the caregiver), and nervous about her ability to accomplish her relational, educational, and medical goals.

Not all of these diverse, tangled, and admittedly, fluctuating factors become evident during health care interactions; not all may be salient to all patients. Yet, the potentiality of these face concerns lurk, in varying forms and magnitudes, for caregivers and their women patients. Further, the multifaceted nature of identities and the diverse possibilities for relational definitions both necessitates facework and complicates it. The lack of singularity—in terms of individual and relational identity—forces the continual reconfiguring of "who are we" and "who are we to each other." Complicating those ongoing hermeneutic and relational undertakings, the interactants must juggle the consequences of those efforts to capture identity and to facilitate face on the fragments of self and relational definitions that are not highlighted at the particular moment in time but that cannot be discarded nor ignored.

The need is clear for ways of engaging in facework wherein women patients and their caregivers may alleviate face threats and accommodate face needs, amidst the complexity and ambiguity of health care interactions and the multiplicity of relational and individual identities and goals. For caregivers and their patients to realize a multidimensional relationship, especially one that encompasses a partnership dimension, they must employ artful means of presenting and affirming each other that make it possible for them to oblige the fragmentation of life and identity in the postmodern era.

Identification

As we have detailed, scholars typically depict health care encounters as inherently asymmetrical encounters (e.g., Davis, 1985, 1988a, 1988b; Fisher, 1984, 1986, 1991, 1993a, 1993b, 1995; Frankel, 1993, 1995; Modaff, 1995;

Todd & Fisher, 1993; West, 1984, 1993a, 1993b). Some dimensions of the emergent caregiver–patient relational system may need to be complementary, perhaps even rigidly so—especially when the caregiver needs to ask for information and the patient needs to provide it. Yet, to foster the realization of both individuals as complex and multifaceted, and to give voice to a multiplicity of identities, caregivers and their patients must co-construct a dynamic in which they may mark their connectedness and demonstrate appreciation of those many relevant identities. We argue that they can do so through *identification.*

In our conceptualization of identification as a relational activity that can contribute to the co-accomplishment of a partnership dimension of health care interactions, we borrow heavily from the writings of Kenneth Burke (1950). Burke contended that shared symbols enable individuals to identify with others, to talk in terms of what both parties know and can understand. As they communicate with each other in light of a particular commonality, individuals mark the mutuality of that portion of their lives, or, as Burke (1950) noted, "in being identified with B, A is 'substantially one' with a person other than himself" (p. 21).

Yet, this concept of "consubstantiality" (see Burke, 1950) does not diminish the potentiality of a multitude of individual or relational identities. According to Burke, "Two persons may be identified in terms of some principle they share in common, an 'identification' that does not deny their distinctness" (p. 21). In so doing, people may achieve identification or connectedness with regard to some aspect of their lives although not disregarding other parts of their relational dynamic, other fragments of their individual identities.

Hence, as caregivers and patients come together, they are thrust into an interactional context wherein they are interrelated and interdependent (see Bateson, 1951; Watzlawick et al., 1967). The emergent co-construction of their relationship is something that is unique because of the combination of the two interactants. However, as we have discussed previously, in light of the postmodern era, that dyad may not be restricted to a monolithic definition. As the interactants struggle to position themselves and to realize their multiplicity of preferred identities, the concept of "identification" has never been more important nor more difficult.

The fragmentation of the postmodern era seems only to enhance Burke's (1950) rationale for the need for identification. In this era, we are not only nomadic travelers, scrambling between links with others, obligations, and ways of viewing the world; we consist of shattered selves, inherently divided within ourselves and in the world. We are simultaneously somewhat connected and somewhat isolated. Burke explained:

In pure identification there would be no strife. Likewise, there would be no strife in absolute separateness, since opponents can join battle only through a mediatory ground that makes their communication possible, thus providing

the first condition necessary for their interchange of blows. But put identification and division ambiguously together, so that you cannot know for certain
just where one ends and the other begins, and you have the characteristic
invitation to rhetoric. (p. 25)

For, in many ways, what we are suggesting here *is* implicitly rhetorical.
Caregivers and their patients must engage in an artful, interactional dance,
where their moves affect all other moves, their identifications necessarily
impact, constrain, and potentially, enrich other identifications. As they advance their own preferences for how they want to be treated (and how they
want to treat their interactional counterparts), they necessarily take part in
interpersonal persuasion. In fact, Burke (1950) proposed that "there is no
chance of our keeping apart the meanings of persuasion, identification ('consubstantiality') and communication (the nature of rhetoric as 'addressed')"
(p. 46).

Although Burke's writings have traditionally been referred to in analyses
of discourse in public forums, we herald the applicability of his work to the
interpersonal context. We believe that his concept of identification depicts
an activity that occurs in everyday life between interactants as they attempt
to co-determine commonalities, to co-establish a common ground for their
interactions. Furthermore, given our postmodern view of relational communication in the health care context, we feel that the idea of identification is
especially salient and important. If we acknowledge the premise that
caregivers and their patients may work toward the co-accomplishment of a
multiplicity of individual and relational identities, and we accept the notion
that the confusion and conflict of the postmodern era precludes static role
and situational definitions, then those caregivers and patients must find some
way of latching on to some at least temporary common ground; they must
grasp some snippet of connectedness, especially in terms of a potential
partnership dimension of their relationship.

Although we recognize that Burke's ideas have been primarily used for
modernist ends (for exemplars of such applications of Burke, see Cheney,
1983; Crable, 1977; Gaines, 1979; Gibson, 1970; Leff, 1973; Sanbonmatsu,
1971), we hold that Burke's ideas also lend themselves to understanding
aspects of communication in the postmodern era as well (see Beck & Aden,
1996; Payne, 1995). Payne contended that Burke's writings have "much in
common with the core of postmodernist thought" (p. 334). Furthermore, Beck
and Aden (1996) provide an exemplar of a postmodern re-reading of Burke
and his concept of identification; they argued that "Burke's writings suggest
an ongoing process of identification as we flirt with multiple identities."

We argue that identification constitutes a significant relational activity,
especially for the co-achievement of a partnership dimension (and reflexively, for other relational activities such as facework) in the health care
context. In the following chapters, we pursue how that relational activity of

identification may be realized as well as the implicativeness of identification for the co-accomplishment of goals.

Interactional Framing

If interactants in health care encounters dabble in a multiplicity of simultaneous relational and individual identities, and if those interactants bring various relational, educational, and medical goals to the encounter, and if those interactants enter the health care encounter with a plethora of possible (and perhaps, even conflicting) expectations, beliefs, understandings, and so on, about "what should go on here" and "how we should act together," then they confront the monumental interactional challenge of discerning—and co-constructing with each other—working definitions about the nature of the situation and their relationship with each other. We believe that it is too easy to look at the structural asymmetry of medical encounters and assume that the doctor controls and that the patient meekly obeys. We do not deny that such "control–obey" relational scenarios occur; we do contend that there is an ever-increasing awareness by health care professionals, health care educators, and patients that caregivers and their patients need to address the multifaceted nature of their relationship and the encounter (see discussion in Chapter 1).

However, the co-achievement of such a dynamic, within the tight time constraints of typical health care encounters, requires caregivers and patients to carefully communicate to each other "what is happening now" and "where do we go from here." We maintain that interactants indicate such temporal, ever-emergent, sign-posting through metacommunicative interactional framing.

Bateson (1951, 1972) introduced the concept of *framing* in his theory of play. Bateson (1951) suggested that participants—his initial study focused on zoo monkeys—somehow frame their interaction. That is, they offer each other signals about how behavior is to be taken (in the case of the monkeys, serious frames vs. play frames; see Bateson, 1951).

In *Frame Analysis*, Goffman (1974) advanced Bateson's theory of framing by describing how metacommunicative cues or "keys" mark how a spate of talk should be construed by fellow interactants. Although Watzlawick et al. (1967) referred to the metacommunicative function of positive and negative feedback for relational systems, Goffman (1974) took a more local view of "keyings" by focusing on how interactants know how talk may be framed, not necessarily the relational implicativeness of that framing. (Despite that concentration, however, Goffman, 1974, did explore the interactional problems with "breaking frame" or behaving out of frame.)

According to Goffman (1974), framework implies that interactants converse in a primary frame for the most part, perhaps based on the central focus of the interaction or their main roles in the encounter. Goffman (1974) contended that interactants may shift out of that frame to engage temporarily in some activity that would not normally fit within the primary frame. Hence, interactants need to offer and interpret cues or keys so that they can contribute to keeping the interaction "on track" and so they can be taken as participating in a manner that fits with their respective stature and part in the conversation.

In many ways, this view of a primary frame dovetails with the work of sociolinguists who maintain that individuals who are competent in multiple cultures behave in a manner that permits them to differentiate between their self-presentation in one culture and not in another one through code-switching (see Ervin-Tripp, 1971; Grimshaw, 1971; Gumperz, 1971). To display their orientation to others (as possible co-members) and to their relationship to others in the interaction, Gumperz maintained that they speak in the "appropriate" code. The interactants distinguish "who we are to each other now" (as opposed to on other occasions) via talking or acting in distinguishable ways (i.e., code-switching). For example, the talk between a manager and an employee may vary from their time in the boardroom to their time on the ballfield. However, Ervin-Tripp (1971) contended that code-switching may be particularly problematic for interactants "where status is clearly specified, speech style is rigidly prescribed, and the form of address of each person is derived from his social identity" (p. 19).

Although Goffman's (1974) conception of framing is more fluid and less dramatic of a shift from one activity to another than the sociolinguists' stance on code-switching, the flaw from a postmodern perspective stems from Goffman's rather monolithic, modernist treatment of what may occur during interactions—in terms of singularity of topic, activity, etc.—and how people demonstrate movement *from* one culture, role, frame, issue, identity, and so on *to* another, seemingly an either–or rather than a both-and model. Research in the health care context that acknowledges a debt to Goffman's work on interactional framing also tends to suffer from a heavily modernist conception of social activity (see Beck & Ragan, 1992; Coyne, 1985; Davies, 1981; Emerson, 1970; Evans, Block, Steinberg, & Penrose, 1986; see also the excellent review of this body of literature in Chenail, 1991).

Although Goffman (1974) certainly referred to the idea of embeddedness in his description of "lamination," the "either–or" dichotomies of frame versus frame resound throughout his book as well as the forenoted works. The problem for researchers, and for everyday interactants as well, is to grapple with the both–and-ness of a multiplicity of simultaneous activities as well as the consequentiality and reflexivity of those activities. Interactants, especially during health care encounters, do not simply do one thing or another (no more than they can be one way or another).

However, just as modernist tendencies hinder caregiver and patient attempts to affirm multiple and diverse identities and goals, a modernist approach to conversation can cover the intertangled nature of conversational topics and activities. As we detail later, caregivers, in particular, routinely succumb to either–or-like moves between topics, ignoring the relatedness and the complicated, interwoven nature of activities, concerns, goals, and identities. Without addressing the both–and-ness, caregivers and patients implicitly don blinders that limit their gaze and isolate out aspects of the broader picture that could be valuable and enlightening. They miss opportunities for perspective.

However, the paradox lies in discerning how interactants can co-accomplish the both–and as opposed to the either–or, how they bracket a snippet of conversation or action as not really fitting within the rest of the simultaneous activity while the instance of bracketing, keying, and so on, works in and of itself, to facilitate and enrich that activity. Given the constant hermeneutic process (see Gadamer, 1975, 1976, 1988) and the consequentiality of verbal and nonverbal behaviors for the interaction and for the relationship (see Watzlawick et al., 1967), we maintain that interactants cannot legitimately just say "time out" and indicate that some action simply does not count or that it must be interpreted as totally unrelated to the business at hand. Although they may indeed attempt to do so, we suggest that relational consequences stem from those denials of some salient dimension of the interaction or the relationship. As Sally told Harry in *When Harry Met Sally*, interactants cannot take anything back, pretend like an event did not happen, or try to write it off as something that is unrelated and nonconsequential to the dyad. In Sally's words, "It's already out there," and it *does* mesh with and impact everything else.

Thus, as we come to this paradox of how interactants tag a bit of talk or an action as different yet as fitting within the interaction (as well as facilitating a multifaceted, complex, relational dynamic), we take the postmodern position that metacommunicative interactional framing can enable interactants to attend to their multiplicity of identities and goals. By re-conceptualizing interactional framing, we can accommodate the both–and-ness of identities, activities, and systemic definitions. We do so by borrowing Goffman's contention that interactants metacommunicatively signal each other about "what is going on here" as well as by relying on Watzlawick et al.'s (1967) view that metacommunication is something that is both a part of the system while transcending it.

In this view of interactional framing, caregivers and patients can opt to avoid shifts from one activity or topic to another, one set of identities to another; instead, they can offer some metacommunicative cue that recognizes that more than one activity is being accomplished here yet one may be highlighted. As we exemplify and detail throughout the rest of this volume, interactional framing involves less of a shift from one dimension to another than a magnification of one aspect of the caregiver and patient's multifaceted relationship.

Reflexive Interplay

Although we explained our perspectives of the relational activities of face-work, identification, and interactional framing separately, we want to emphasize the reflexivity of those activities. In some of our earlier writings (see Beck & Ragan, 1992, 1995; Ragan, Beck, & White, 1995), we took a rather linear approach to these activities, suggesting uni-directionally, for example, that identification may lead to facework in health care interactions. In so doing, we seemed to place "facework" at the top of some hierarchy without appreciating the potentiality of the reverse nor of the interplay between these two relational activities. As we look back on that work and forward to the current one from a postmodern perspective, we realize that "facework" is intricately interwoven with other relational activities, augmenting them and becoming possible through them.

The activities of facework, identification, and interactional framing work reflexively throughout caregiver–patient interactions. Certainly, when caregivers and patients co-accomplish identification (and in so doing, co-establish a common ground, perhaps as fellow women, fellow professionals, partners), that activity of identification simultaneously involves (as well as makes possible) facework. Identification with regard to one dimension of their relational dynamic absolutely impacts countless other aspects of their respective individual and relational identities and goals (i.e., the caregiver could inadvertently affirm, disconfirm, reify, or undermine other identities that drift just beyond the superficies).

Similarly, facework can reflexively facilitate identification. Through face-work, caregivers and their patients can avoid embarrassment and achieve preferred face as well as nurture fertile soil for the springing forth demonstrations of—and referrals to—likeness, similarities, potentially with regard to a multiplicity of relational identities. Furthermore, interactional framing enables caregivers and patients to mark attention to pieces of fragmented relational and individual identity, again both encompassing and providing the means through which caregivers and patients may co-achieve facework and identification.

This reflexive nature of relational activities necessitates an orientation to facework, identification, and interactional framing as interdependent and mutually reifying, not as a linear process wherein one leads to the other without reciprocation, not in terms of a hierarchy of significance. Furthermore, the reflexive interplay of these activities works concurrently to facilitate how the relationship ensues, how the caregiver and the patient collaborate to intermingle (or interactionally ignore) the multiplicity of possible relational and individual identities, and importantly, relational, medical, and educational goals.

REFLEXIVITY OF CONVERSATIONAL ACTIVITIES

As we have been suggesting throughout this book, caregivers and patients come to health care encounters as complicated individuals, their selves fragmented by a scattered collection of diverse yet interconnected identities. At the most basic level, a caregiver and patient enter the room to accomplish the giving and receiving of care. If the caregiver and patient are to establish a partnership, though, their involvement with each other must facilitate the realization of the multiplicity of identities beyond just one person with a problem and one person with possible solutions. Instead, they must co-discover how their diverse and multifaceted identities fit together, overlapping and complementing; they must co-achieve a relational dynamic wherein preferred individual and relational identities are facilitated not ignored, nurtured not damaged. Although their individual and relational identities are fluid and ever-developing, caregivers and patients can commence mutual understanding by acknowledging the overwhelming complexity and multidimensional nature of each other and their relationship. In so doing, they start to piece together chips of the puzzle. Although they perpetually seek tiny, elusive bits, they can begin to see forms and outlines of at least one dimension of the evolving picture.

The process necessarily involves a collaborative effort wherein the multiplicity of identities—of both caregiver and patient—must be appreciated and recognized, not assumed to be checked at the door before the health care visit commences. Through their relational communication, through the reflexive nature of their verbal and nonverbal actions, choice of activities, and so on, caregivers and patients co-determine how they will relate to each other and what they will treat as important and relevant. We argue that interactants can artfully acknowledge the multiplicity of relational and individual identities, thus facilitating face and identification relational activities as well as preferred relational definitions, via intimating that multiplicity during their conversations.

Given our micro-analytic position that interactants co-accomplish numerous, diverse activities during their conversations as well as our view that the reflexivity of language permits such simultaneous co-occurence of activities, our task now is to examine how caregivers and patients may coordinate their behaviors in order to display and co-achieve preferred individual and relational identities as well as other educational and medical goals. For the remainder of this chapter, we focus on the collaborative co-achievement of individual and relational identities. We believe that those identities underlie yet also include other relational goals that focus on the emergent relationship between caregivers and patients.

Although we cannot reach inside the minds of the interactants to discern their cognitive states, their internal goals, we can pursue how they display preferences for relational dynamics, for treatment of themselves and of the other. We can gain an understanding of how caregivers and patients reciprocatively, reflexively, engage in nonverbal and verbal behaviors that work to advance and affirm (or disconfirm) preferences for how they do (and do not) want to be treated in relation to each other and preferences for what will (and will not) occur (i.e., the ongoing, always temporal, always incomplete, co-definition of complex, fluid systemic boundaries and rules) through conversational activities.

In particular, we explore the achievement (as well as the reflexive nature) of, first, affirmation of a multiplicity of patient identities (via recognition of the patient's opinion, humorous acknowledgment of paradoxes with patient identities, and nonmedical task talk and allusions to commonalities) and, second, affirmation of a multiplicity of caregiver identities (via caregiver personal disclosures). As we observe, the treatment of each of the participants as complex, multidimensional individuals works reflexively to facilitate the realization of a multiplicity of relational identities, especially a partner-partner like dynamic. Additionally, we explain how caregivers and patients can co-accomplish those conversational activities without elongating medical interviews nor ignoring necessary medical tasks.

Affirmation of Multiplicity of Patient Identities

As explained earlier, patients confront the paradox of wanting to bring their plethora of voices to the health care visit while simultaneously not knowing how to do so, when to do so, or what is appropriate to share. Certainly, not all aspects of an individual's cornucopia of fragmented identities emerge during any single interaction with another person; however, for a partnership aspect of a relationship between a patient and a caregiver to ensue during health care encounters, the patient must be recognized and treated as more than "just a patient" for numerous reasons.

A strict focus on the patient as simply a person with medical concerns puts that patient in an inherently complementary role to caregiver: The caregiver directs the interaction to assess the nature of the problem; because that patient has solicited the input of this individual with medical expertise, the patient enables the caregiver to determine the problem and to recommend solutions. In such an asymmetrical model, the caregiver and patient minimize the likelihood of a partner–partner relationship because the patient is treated as someone who brings little more than a problem to the encounter.

When the caregiver *and* the patient fail to collaboratively refer to the patient as complex and multifaceted, they do not permit acknowledgment of the multiple identities that can make the patient a viable partner; they ignore the diversity of the patient's experience, understanding, and perspective; they diagnose the concern with the body in isolation of the multiplicity of identities that use that body as a vessel, not a definition. However, given 10 minutes, given complicated medical tasks, given varying, perhaps conflicting, fragments of knowledge, expectations, and preconceptions, the notion of treating the whole person is daunting. We suggest that a way to make the multiplicity of patient identities relevant is to make brief references to those identities, not to pursue each in depth, marking each that is tapped lightly as *an* identity without necessarily lingering on any of them as *the* one defining identity.

This process entails an artful balance of doing more recognizing than ignoring, more affirming than disconfirming, more encouraging than discouraging, more empowering than sugar-coating, more identifying than alienating on the part of both caregivers and patients. Given the complexity and multiplicity of identities and goals, each of these will likely occur to some extent, and none are necessarily even "good" or "bad." Yet the co-accomplishment of facework and identification as well as individual and relational identities depends on the interactants striking a collaborative equilibrium between (and co-definition of) these ways of responding to each other.

Recognition of Patient Opinions. In Excerpts 2, 7, and 8, a female medical doctor meets with an adolescent female. This doctor believes that teens should be examined without their parents present so that they may raise issues that they may not want to discuss in front of their parents. In so doing, the doctor implicitly demonstrates her initial perspective on teens as young adults who should have privacy and who should take part as individuals (not just as "children") in dialogues with health care professionals (similar to Linda, the nurse at the beginning of this chapter). Notably, the doctor does not ignore the facts that these teens are minors and that each is someone's child. Instead, she opts to highlight another aspect of the identities of teens that could be easily swept under the rug if she permitted their parents to accompany them in the examining room.

In "Michelle's" case, the caregiver (C) attends to a medical complaint while also voicing awareness and appreciation of the patient's (P) family situation. In so doing, she also alludes to prior interactions with Michelle and Michelle's family. When we examine very micro details of the talk between the caregiver and Michelle, we incorporate some of the transcription notations that were developed by Gail Jefferson (see Atkinson & Heritage, 1984; please see Appendix B for a description of these notations).

Excerpt 2:

1   C: Are you blowing a lot of the clear stuff?
2   P: Yeah, it's clear.
3   C: Okay, so it's not real thick yellow stuff.

4	P:	mm mm
5	C:	Do you feel a lot of pressure in your sinus=
6	P:	=It hurts all right in here. And my ear'll start hurtin
7		right in here sometimes.
8	C:	Okay, so it is hurtin up in=
9	P:	=and my head hurts all in here.
10	C:	Okay. It sounds like something. You probably are gettin
11		a sinus infection. Are you coughin any?
12	P:	Yeah, I was earlier=
13	C:	=so=
14	P:	=and my throat was itching and coughing
15	C:	okay=
16	P:	=a lot

In Excerpt 2, the doctor and Michelle discuss the specific symptoms that Michelle has been experiencing. Certainly, the doctor asks questions, and Michelle gives answers; however, this example of medical talk also reveals a collaborative effort in which their emergent relational system may not be simply characterized as "complementary."

For example, this doctor offers a number of acknowledgments of Michelle's description of her condition. In lines 8, 10, and 15, the doctor responds to the Michelle's statements with "okay." In lines 8 and 10, the doctor continues with her turn at talk by repeating Michelle's claim of pain (line 8) and by affirming her problem by noting that "it sounds like something" and voicing a possible diagnoses—a "sinus infection" (lines 10 and 11). In so doing, the doctor treats Michelle as a person who can speak for herself and who has legitimate concerns. (Notably, the doctor also positions herself as someone who can draw that conclusion—the "expert" part of her identity.)

Additionally, Michelle's utterances during the conversation work to position her as an active co-participant. In lines 2 and 4, she refrains her responses to direct answers to the doctor's questions; however, in lines 6 and 7, she asserts her description beyond the narrow focus of the doctor's question. Although the doctor asks about Michelle's sinus, Michelle stresses that she does not simply feel pressure in her sinus. She contends, "It hurts all right in here," and she continues by noting the pain in her ear. The caregiver begins to acknowledge that hurt; however, Michelle breaks in again by adding that "and my head hurts all in here."

Although these interactants are very much engaged in "medical talk," they necessarily, simultaneously, communicate relationally. Through her responses to Michelle, the doctor implicitly displays her awareness of Michelle as not just a child, not just someone with symptoms, not just someone who has come for care or treatment. The doctor gathers information in a manner that marks respect for Michelle's input, for example, accepting Michelle's descriptions, permitting Michelle to take the lead in offering more details. The doctor does so while still presenting herself as an "expert" (see her tentative diagnosis in lines 10 and 11) and as someone who can move from acknowledgments of Michelle's responses to then ask further questions (see line 11). The doctor gives nothing away with regard to her own multiplicity of identities by empowering Michelle to be more than just a person with a problem.

Michelle reflexively treats the doctor as someone who permits her to speak up and to participate without ramifications. Some may contend that, as a teen, Michelle may just be at the age where she will talk without regard for authority or where she has not been exposed to the mix of cultural preconceptions about doctor–patient interaction. We accept those contentions as possibilities. However, we suggest here that the doctor and the patient contributed to the collaborative co-achievement of a relational dynamic wherein such assertions may occur, regardless of the patient's age.

If the doctor had interrupted Michelle's assertions or disregarded them, either on this occasion or during prior interactions, then the doctor would have disconfirmed the participant aspect of the patient's preferred set of individual identities. Such a snub would have been consequential to how the interaction then ensued as well as to how the two could converse in the future. If the doctor had responded to Michelle's assertions by marking them as a sort of threat to some chunk of the doctor's collage of identities, that response would have served as what Watzlawick et al. (1967) dubbed "positive feedback," promoting change in the proposed system. Because the doctor opted to affirm (instead of disconfirm) and because the patient chose to assert (instead of simply to answer), the nature of their talk about a medical concern permitted them to reflexively co-accomplish an emergent relational dynamic wherein such participation is acceptable.

For example, in Excerpt 3, the female doctor interacts with a new patient whom we will call "Susan." The patient's health insurance plan changed so she comes to this new physician seeking continued care for an ongoing health concern. Interestingly, Susan begins overtly by stating her agenda for the encounter, to get a specific prescription instead of to seek the doctor's input on what a correct or appropriate drug might be. Although the very approach that Susan takes serves to position her definitively as a consumer and a participant, it also could be construed by the doctor as threatening to aspects of her own face, such as her self-presentation as "expert."

Excerpt 3:

1   C: Well, what brought you in today?
2   P: Ummm, I would like a prescription for Annaprox or Colestol=
3   C: =uhh huh=

4	P:	=I had a, I used to have, I've had both of those in the
5		past, and they're fine, and the last doctor at the clinic
6		gave me Nephafalod, and I don't think it's as effective=
7	C:	=huh=
8	P:	=And I don't know what it's supposed to do, cause
9		[I never (unintelligible)]
10	C:	[I think] that's probably just the generic of Neclon
11		[I bet]
12	P:	[What is that] supposed to do? Is it the same thing as
13		it doesn't seem to work as [well to me]
14	C:	[as Annaprox?]=
15	P:	=naahh
16	C:	[yeah, now]
17	P:	[nah]=
18	C:	=see=
19	P:	=It doesn't seem to stop the pain=
20	C:	=Tell me about what it's what all this is for
21	P:	umm, menstrual cramps=
22	C:	=ohh okay and=
23	P:	=um=
24	C:	=Annaprox works better.
25	P:	Annaprox and Postol they both work about the same=
26	C:	=yeah=
27	P:	=and they stop the pain which is really [critical for me]
28	C:	[ohh sure]=
29	P:	=and um and that stuff=
30	C:	yeah [you know]
31	P:	[it] it dulls it somewhat [but]
32	C:	[but] it doesn't work
33		as well=
34	P:	=noo=
35	C:	=that's interesting yeah they're all in the same class=
36	P:	=unh=
37	C:	they're all anti-inflammatories=
38	P:	=uh huh=
39	C:	=there's probably like thirty different anti-inflammatories=
40	P:	=huh=
41	C:	=and in my experience some one [a given]
42	P:	[uh huh]
43	C:	One will work better for one patient, and another one will
44		work [better] for another
45	P:	[yeah]
46	C:	so I bet that the reason whoever gave you this did was

```
47          because=
48    P:    =it's just=
49    C:    =for for a long time this one was sort of touted as being
50          one of the best for menstrual cramps=
51    P:    =huh=
52    C:    =but I use either Motrin or the Annaprox=
53    P:    =uh huh=
54    C:    =it's um yeah=
55    P:    =umm
56    C:    so no I sure don't have a problem [with that]
57    P:                                      [okay]
```

Without describing symptoms or identifying a medical problem, Susan expresses her desire for "Annaprox or Colestol" in line 2. The doctor acknowledges her request (line 3), and Susan then proceeds to give an account for why she wants either of those drugs—she received a prescription for another medication from a previous doctor, and it "doesn't seem to work as well to me" (lines 4–6, 8–9, 12–13).

Although the doctor still has no idea about the medical necessity that Susan has for such a drug, she enables her to continue after her initial request by saying "uhh huh" in line 3. Furthermore, she does not criticize Susan's analysis of the effectiveness of Nephafalod nor does she attempt to interject her own opinion at this point. She merely says "huh" in line 7, offers a clarification of the drug in lines 10–11, and prompts a comparison of Nephafalod and Annaprox in line 14.

Only after Susan's agreement ("naahh") that the doctor is correct in her clarification that Annaprox is the drug that is being compared to Nephafalod, the doctor attempts to gain the floor in lines 16 and 18, with one more interjection by Susan that the latter "doesn't seem to stop the pain." At that point, the doctor finally asks why the patient has the pain in line 20.

Throughout this portion of conversation, the doctor permits Susan to offer her opinion; she does not deny Susan's view of the drugs or how they work in her body. Furthermore, upon learning the reason for Susan's need for medication (menstrual cramps), she ratifies Susan's perspective that "Annaprox works better" (line 24). Interestingly, Susan then observes that "Annaprox and Postol [not a drug on her list of choices at the outset] they both work about the same." The doctor affirms Susan's knowledge of the drugs yet she also goes on to advance her own expertise by noting that a whole class of anti-inflammatories exists (lines 35, 37, and 39) and by referring to her experience (line 41).

However, again, she does so in a way that does not take away from Susan's self-positioning as an informed person, a consumer, a person in pain with her own set of experiences. In fact, in lines 43 and 44, the doctor

recognizes the validity of Susan's observations as well as the uniqueness of
every case by remarking "one will work better for one patient, and another
one will work better for another." After reiterating her understanding of the
drugs in question by suggesting a possible rationale for Susan's last prescription in lines 46–47 and 49–50, the doctor informs Susan that the Annaprox is one of her own drugs of choice. The way in which the doctor
sets up this admission (as well as the granting of the patient's request) allows
her to do so as an expert, not just as someone who simply "gives in" without
cause. It also reflexively gives credence to Susan's own convictions about
the value and usefulness of this particular drug for her specific case, thus
affirming parts of Susan's multidimensional collection of identities (i.e.,
knowledgeable consumer, active patient) which she opted to make relevant
at the outset of the interaction.

In Excerpt 4, though, a female nurse practitioner confronts the challenge
of dealing with the face needs of a patient who has inaccurate information.
The nurse practitioner is a health caregiver at a university health care facility;
the patient is a young female university student ("Nancy") who expresses a
concern about her irregular periods and a desire for a Pap smear.

Excerpt 4:

```
 1   C:   mm kay well >you really don't< need another Pap smear now
 2        (.)
 3   P:   Aren't >cha sposed ta< have um >evry six months<? (.)
 4   C:   no:o (.) once a year=
 5   P:   oh that's what >somebody told me<=
 6   C:   oh no >once a [year,]
 7   P:                 [>it's why<] I come in cuz I don want=
 8   C:   =well let me see [what]=
 9   P:                    [(indistinguishable)]
10   C:   =your last hhh hhh >ya don wanta take< any chances huh?=
11        =[hhh]
12   P:    [hhh] (.)
13   C:   let me see what your last Pap smear showed okay? (.) if you
14        had it in December (.) you won't need another Pap smear
15   P:   okay (.)
16   C:   um:m (.) tha Pap smear waz fine
17   P:   okay
18   C:   um:m (.) hhh we can do >one if you< want hhh one [hhh]
19   P:                                                    [hhh]
20        >that's okay< hhh
21   C:   uh:h (.) >you'll pass< hhh huh? (.) um (.) no (.) what we
22        can do is (.) uh >you know< you might just (.) your body
23        >trying to readjust to these pills< (hhh) now one thing=
```

After the nurse practitioner tells her that she does not "need another Pap smear now," Nancy questions that assessment by offering her belief that she should have one "every six months." As in Excerpts 2 and 3, the expression of patient opinions impacts the co-achievement of individual and relational identities. Those opinions (as well as the way in which the interactants collaboratively co-produce their integration into the conversation) have implications on complex, multifaceted face issues. Unlike the previous two excerpts however, this caregiver disagrees with the opinion of the patient regarding her medical needs.

The expression and recognition of patient opinions can constitute a potential face threat to caregivers. In this case, the query poses a direct challenge to the nurse practitioner's knowledge because it marks the nurse practitioner's reading of Nancy's file as perhaps incorrect. Nancy does not say "I know that you are wrong" or "I have better information"; she chooses a less direct path. However, whether stated indirectly or directly, her question makes the disparity in beliefs and information a problematic issue for the emergent conversation and relational dynamic. Reflexively, the fact that Nancy asks such a question also contributes to the co-definition of who she is and how she wants to be treated. It enables her to advance fragments of her preferred face (i.e., as someone who has knowledge, who wants to participate in her health care, who prefers to be taken as an active consumer, who has viable, real health care concerns).

After hearing the nurse practitioner state hesitantly yet deliberately that Pap smears should be conducted "once a year" (line 4), Nancy pursues the issue by noting that "somebody told me" that she should have one, bringing some outside, unnamed, implied expert into the conversation as support (line 5). The nurse practitioner reiterates her stance by saying "oh no >once a year<" (line 6). At that point, Nancy overtly emphasizes that the reason for her visit is the Pap smear, not simply her irregular periods (line 7).

To continue the "no, you don't–yes, I do" circle of arguments, the nurse practitioner and her patient could have started a downward spiral, resulting in threats to the nurse practitioner's face as an expert and to the patient's face as an involved, knowledgeable consumer, a person with significant health concerns. Instead, the nurse practitioner moves out of the circle by agreeing to take another look at the patient's chart, to re-check her assessment of the patient's need for the Pap smear (line 8). In so doing, the nurse practitioner acknowledges her own potential fallibility, and in so doing, she sets up a situation where the primary determinant for the final decision becomes the result of Nancy's last Pap smear, not the nurse practitioner's perspective, not Nancy's opinion.

As the nurse practitioner shifts their attention to Nancy's chart (beginning in line 8), she interjects a metacommunicative acknowledgment of a possible reason for Nancy to want the Pap smear. After all, Pap smears involve an uncomfortable process that most women dislike and even dread. For Nancy to assert herself in this manner, she must have some reason, possibly a combination of conflicting grounds, convictions, and fears, stemming from assorted life experiences and pieces of information. Because Nancy insists on something that other women—likely even herself—disprefer and because she is arguing with the nurse practitioner, and so on, Nancy gets tangled in a face-threatening paradox: Do not insist and maybe die *or* do insist and risk appearing rude or odd.

In line 10, the nurse practitioner interrupts herself midthought to verbally recognize what would be a reasonable rationale for Nancy to behave as she does: "ya don wanta take any chances huh," followed by a brief laugh. In so doing, the nurse practitioner indicates to Nancy that she understands Nancy's apprehension and persistence, that it makes sense to her. The laughter (which is shared by Nancy) potentially addresses the paradox—the patient's concern about this form of preventative screening is simultaneously viable yet unnecessary, consistent with parts of her goals and identities yet inconsistent with others—as well as Nancy's possible embarrassment because of that paradox. Through her acknowledgment of Nancy's motivation for obtaining a Pap smear, the nurse practitioner also meta-recognizes the tension and awkwardness of the preceding moments of the interaction as well as at least part of Nancy's face needs.

In lines 13 through 14, the nurse practitioner gains Nancy's agreement that they will let the last Pap smear indicate the necessity of a present one. After the nurse practitioner tells Nancy that "tha Pap smear was <u>fine</u>" (line 16), Nancy drops her pursuit of the test. The nurse practitioner gives her one last chance to request the Pap smear, but the nurse practitioner does so jokingly, indicating her levity by laughing. As noted by a number of students of conversation and humor, laughter is sequentially implicative; that is, interactants cue each other with regard to preferences for treating utterances through the placement of laughables and laughter (see Glenn, 1989; Jefferson, 1979, 1984; Sacks, 1974). In this second laughter sequence (lines 18–21), Nancy does respond with brief laughs after the nurse practitioner begins to laugh first, thus marking the prior utterance as a potential laughable. Although the nurse practitioner attempts to extend the laughter sequence in line 21 with "you'll pass hhh huh?", Nancy does not reciprocate. The nurse practitioner continues with her turn—albeit hesitantly and disfluently—and redirects the conversation back to the original problem before the discussion of the Pap smear, Nancy's concern about irregular periods.

As we discuss in the next portion of this chapter, humorous acknowledgments of paradoxes with patient identity can facilitate facework as well as identification between caregivers and patients. However, in this particular case, although such a lighthearted reference might be appropriate to some parts of Nancy's identity (i.e., the woman who likely would not enjoy such an examination), we wonder whether or not such laughter also may have worked to undermine other fragments of Nancy's identity—the consumer, the concerned patient. The laughter could well have intensified the paradox.

Given the nurse practitioner's laughter, her prior conviction that Nancy does not need a Pap smear, and inference that the exam is something that Nancy would "want" as opposed to something that is medically necessary, could Nancy still legitimately have asked for a Pap smear without feeling even more inconsistent with how "reasonable" women might act? Although Nancy again shares the nurse practitioner's laughter and says "that's okay" to the invitation, we have no information available (nor does the caregiver) that would suggest Nancy's level of satisfaction with the encounter and with the unattained goal of obtaining a Pap smear. We do not know whether Nancy was convinced that a Pap smear was not really necessary.

Although the nurse practitioner did engage in facework by a recognition of Nancy's desire not to take "any chances," the usefulness of the second effort at appreciating Nancy's opinion is less clear. Earlier, Beck and Ragan suggested that "if P [patient] is still truly concerned, she now has an opportunity to request a Pap smear without again losing face. Further, NP [nurse practitioner] invites P to join her in shared laughter about the idea of a Pap smear . . ." (1992, p. 57).

As we look at this excerpt now, in light of our ideal of the co-creation of a partnership-like dynamic, we contend that the invitation might have served a face-saving function. However, to treat the patient as a partner (and as a multifaceted person who has her own assortment of knowledge, her own diverse beliefs, her own scattered experiences and interactions and desires), we feel that the invitation may have worked better as a process of information evaluation in which the nurse practitioner could have collaborated with the patient to determine her underlying fears and the reasons for her beliefs and to share medical knowledge and perspectives.

The nurse practitioner and Nancy looked at the issue as a "yes or no" one in terms of whether Pap smears should or should not be conducted every 6 months. Even if the nurse practitioner was "right," and the patient was "wrong," however, Nancy never received new information to replace her old information about the medical rationale for the timing of the examination. Nancy was encouraged to trust in her old Pap smear test and in the nurse practitioner's expertise (and thus, to distrust her own instincts and understanding) without substantial grounds for doing so.

Furthermore, the nurse practitioner did not seek, nor did the patient offer, details about the patient's lived reality. By not treating the situation as gray and murky (instead of clear and certain), the nurse practitioner could not truly enable that patient to sort through complex and conflicting ideas and issues, to make good choices for her, as a multidimensional individual.

Did Nancy have a choice in this case? We believe that the "invitation" was offered and treated as a nicety—a laughable, not a legitimate alternative to consider, because it lacked a sincere expression of support and understanding by the nurse practitioner. That choice was dubbed laughable, not viable. For Nancy, the face risk of defying conventional medical wisdom and her caregiver as well as potentially contradicting parts of herself could have been too great for her to pursue her medical goal of obtaining the examination and her relational goal of becoming a true participant, a partner, in her health care decisions.

Verbal recognition of patient opinions can affirm aspects of patient perspectives during health care interactions. However, as we have observed throughout this section, such acknowledgment of the patient works reflexively to facilitate the realization of a multiplicity of patient identities and the achievement of a complex relational dynamic between caregivers and patients. Verbal recognitions of patient opinions by caregivers do not just make patients "feel good," nor do they undermine caregiver expertise. This dyadic attention to patient perspectives impacts, shapes, and enriches the dyadic system, especially in terms of a potential partnership–collaborative dynamic.

Humorous Acknowledgment of Paradoxes of Patient Identity. As we noted in Excerpt 4, the clash between incongruent, seemingly incompatible goals and fragmented identities can produce paradoxes for patients. In the exchange between the nurse practitioner and the patient, as in everyday life, the face issues were complex and intertwined. To accomplish one set of face needs and relational goals, the patient needed to sublimate other concurrent yet disparate face needs and relational goals. Yet paradoxically, although she might have wanted to accommodate those incompatible aspects of her multifaceted identity, she could not; although she might have wanted to hush the cries of parts of herself that were being threatened or ignored, she could not stifle them; no part of herself could be thrust into irrelevance yet no part of herself could be solely relevant.

In the perpetual both-and-ness of identity and interaction in the postmodern era, individuals struggle with continual dilemmas, but they do so without victory. To affirm one aspect of identity often encompasses a disconfirmation of another; yet because fragments interweave and mesh together, "faceness," by necessity, is a blur of the composite. Similar to our argument in the preceding section, we suggest here that caregivers and patients may deal with implicit paradoxes of identity by bringing them to the forefront instead of shoving them aside. In particular, humor can function as an interactional means through which the paradoxes may be acknowledged, and, although a threat to part of face may still ensue, the intensity is defused—although not eliminated—through this process of joint commiseration.

For example, as Ragan (1990, p. 74) observed, laughter constitutes a way for caregivers and patients to "redress the potential face threat" of gynecologic examinations (see descriptions and analysis in Beck & Ragan, 1992, 1995; Ragan, 1990; Ragan, Beck, & White, 1995). In Excerpt 5, the same female nurse practitioner as in Excerpt 4 is conducting a pelvic examination of another student ("Mandy") at the university health care facility.

Excerpt 5:

```
 1   C:   are you doin okay?
 2   P:   he heh heh alright yeah::: (2.7)
 3   C:   NOT always the best thing to do is it
 4   P:   heh heh [heh (a lit]tle)
 5   C:           [NEVER (just the) thing to spend your after[noon]
 6   P:                              [heh heh heh]          heh [heheh]
 7        I can think of a lot of other things heh heh heh
 8   C:                        heh heh heh oh yes:
 9   P:   definitely=
10   C:   =heh heh heh heh
```

After the nurse practitioner asks her if she is "doin okay" (line 1), Mandy chuckles and says "yeah:::" (line 2). In so doing, Mandy alludes to the conundrum—yes, within the grand scheme of life, she is "doin okay," but examinations certainly are not fun (nor even funny). Yet, Mandy laughs, perhaps pointing to the absurdity of the question—there is no way to *really* be "okay" when this procedure is being done. However, she is not *not* "okay," if she accepts the nature of the examination, an exam that entails invasion of private space, awkward physical probing, disconcerting casting aside—though not being able to totally cast aside—of preferences for self-presentation, for control, for dignity. Because of medical necessity, she can rationalize putting herself in this vulnerable situation, but she cannot transcend those circumstances nor the fragments of herself that it inherently threatens. The "yeah" must be put in the quotation marks of laughter—an implicit "okay but . . ."

The key here is that the nurse practitioner attends to the patient's allusion to multiple realities —"okay" *and* "okay but"—by extending the laughter through adding a laughable ("NOT always the *best thing* to do is it") in line 3. Because the description "best" likely could never appropriately depict this exam as a choice of desirable activities, the nurse practitioner acknowledges the patient's perspective and identifies with it as a fellow woman who knows, a caregiver who understands. With Mandy's treatment of the nurse practitioner's utterance as a laughable, Mandy and the nurse practitioner perpetuate their collaborative co-orientation to the exam as dispreferred and their recognition of the paradox—not the "best thing to do" yet the "thing" that must occur—while, simultaneously, continuing the examination.

In line 5, the nurse practitioner emphasizes that pelvic examinations are "NEVER" the way "to spend your afternoon," reiterating her own comment from line 3 and extending the sequence of laughables. By presenting pelvic examinations as not something that anyone would submit to unless it was necessary, the nurse practitioner offers Mandy an "out" for her current situation—Mandy *has* to be there; she would not *opt* to be. Mandy affirms the laughable and offers line 7 as her own continuation of the shared laughter "I can think of a lot of other things" and re-emphasizes that perspective with "definitely" in line 9. In so doing, the two diffuse the potential face threat to Mandy while simultaneously, reflexively, co-achieving identification—we both understand; we both realize the awkwardness of the situation; we are mutually "in on" and co-constructing the running joke about something that is not funny, not a joke.

As Excerpt 6 indicates as well, co-constructed sequences of shared laughter do more than divert attention from an invasive procedure. Shared laughter between interactants in both Excerpts 5 and 6 reflexively facilitates the co-accomplishment of common orientations to the conversation, to the references of the laughables, to the examination, to the paradox of preference for the exam as well as to "what is going on here" through that conversation and those references. In Excerpt 6, the female nurse practitioner at the university health care facility completes a pelvic examination on another student, "Melissa."

Excerpt 6:

```
1    C:    all done (2.4) thats it (3.5)
2    P:    hhh gee that waz fun [(.1) heh heh heh heh] heh heh (1.2)
3    C:                                [heh heh heh heh heh]
4    C:    oh you wanna do it again? heh heh heh heh=
5    P:    =heh heh heh (.)
6    C:    okay so I'll run all this stuff to the lab
```

After a somewhat lengthy pause at the conclusion of the pelvic examination, Melissa advances the potential laughable "hhh gee that waz fun" in line 2. The nurse practitioner treats Melissa's utterance as a laughable by laughing immediately after "fun" (line 3). Melissa continues to laugh slightly more than the nurse practitioner. After a brief pause (1.2), the nurse practitioner attempts to extend the laughter sequence by asking "oh you wanna do it again?" and then laughing in line 4.

Through humor, Melissa ends a period of silence. She also overtly acknowledges the awkwardness of the examination by referring to it as "fun." After acknowledging Melissa's laughable, the nurse practitioner extends it by offering a potential laughable that resembles Melissa's in terms of sarcasm (similar to the continual reference to examinations as the "thing" throughout the laughables in Excerpt 5).

Notably, the query about Melissa wanting to "do it again" is also similar to the nurse practitioner's question to her patient, Nancy in Excerpt 4. We suggest that the difference here stems from the positioning of the utterance. In Excerpt 6, the potential laughable came as an extension in a series of laughables initiated by the patient. The examination had ended, and no logical reason existed for another one—surely, the suggestion that the patient would want one *must* be a joke. In Excerpt 4, the nurse practitioner offered the question or invitation as a potential laughable immediately after the patient hesitantly deferred to the nurse practitioner. The problem in Excerpt 4 is that the question or invitation intensified the paradox for the patient (treating the invitation as serious had identity and goal consequences; treating it as humorous had identity and goal consequences). Whereas Melissa would not have a reason to agree, Nancy could have wanted to do so. Thus, the attempt at levity in Excerpt 4 may not have been a viable acknowledgment of Nancy's perspective; it might have magnified the gulf between the interactants instead of bridging it, as in Excerpts 5 and 6.

The co-constructed sequences of shared laughter in Excerpts 5 and 6 reflexively facilitate facework by addressing (albeit not eliminating) paradoxes of identity with which patients struggle, especially during gynecologic examinations. Furthermore, as these caregivers and patients collaboratively co-define utterances as laughable, they reciprocally display their co-orientation to the nature of the conversation as well as to the emergent relational dynamic. The shared laughter permits the co-marking of identification in terms of some aspects of their respective selves—for example, "we share this view of this experience," "we identify with each other," despite differing medical parts in the co-achievement of the activity (one conducting an examination, one undergoing an examination). Through the shared laughter, they meta-transcend, although not escape, their strict medical roles to build identification with regard to other simultaneous fragments of their identities.

As caregivers and patients initiate and respond to laughables, they indicate to each other their orientation to the utterances in question, thus engaging in the interactional framing of them. However, that frame must not be viewed as a rigidly distinct relational portrait that hangs in its own gallery; instead, it must be treated as part of a collage of pictures that are intricately interdependent. The interactants engage in verbal play but not just play, not merely random frolic without interactional or relational consequence. Through their ability to tag a segment of talk as one in which laughter may legitimately occur, they reflexively, collaboratively, co-accomplish a bit of conversation that makes sense to both interactants. In addition, that framing of laughter sequences provides caregivers and patients with the necessary co-orientation for the concurrent relational activities of facework and identification to occur. (Notably, however, facework and identification reflexively permit caregivers and patients to perpetuate the ongoing, artful interactional framing; these activities are reciprocally interdependent and invariably linked.)

Although the instances of humor that we discussed in this section involved the gynecologic examination, we stress the applicability of humor to other women's health contexts. By employing humor to acknowledge paradoxes in identities and/or goals, patients may be afforded a forum for expressing—perhaps even bemoaning—their conflicts and their confusion. Humor can enable caregivers and patients to co-produce an interactional context wherein those disparities are voiced and face threats to fragments of self are recognized, although not necessarily resolved. Unless caregivers learn about patient paradoxes, they cannot offer alternatives; they cannot help their patients to discover both–and-like solutions instead of either–or dilemmas.

Nonmedical Task Talk/Allusions to Commonalities. Verbal recognition and humorous acknowledgment of patient perspectives permits patients to integrate diverse parts of themselves into the interaction; however, those conversational activities stem primarily from discussions of or reactions to medical tasks (i.e., doing a diagnosis, doing an assessment of appropriate medication, doing an examination). As we have emphasized throughout this volume, the multidimensional individual cannot be splintered into components such as the "medical" part and the "social" part, the "patient" versus the "professional" versus the "family member" versus the "consumer." To attend to the multiplicity of patient identities, we suggest that references to the multiplicity should be interwoven throughout the interaction, not compartmentalized into the "it's relational–personal time" segment. To do so, interactants would unnecessarily elongate the interaction and limit the potential for understanding implications of interrelationships between identities, especially in terms of medical and educational goals and possible outcomes. By engaging in nonmedical task talk throughout encounters during examinations and discussions of issues, the interactants provide fertile ground for the heralding of commonalities and, thus, the advancement of a partnership-like dynamic.

In Excerpt 7, the female doctor continues her conversation with and examination of Michelle, the teen from Excerpt 2. As they talk, they integrate yet another dimension of Michelle's identity into the interaction. Notably, the doctor begins this portion of their talk while starting the actual physical examination.

Excerpt 7:

17   C: Okay. Well, let's just check you out and see (.1)
18   what's going on. Well how's school going, Michelle?

```
19   P:   Oh, pretty good this year.
20   C:   Is it okay?
21   P:   yeah
22   C:   What grade are you in?
23   P:   Ninth
24   C:   Oh, that's good (.63) Okay. Well, your lungs sound good.
25        Let's see if we can look at your nose and throat (.5)
```

As the doctor starts to examine Michelle (line 17), she references an aspect of Michelle's life that has little to do with the medical task at hand—school (line 18). Notably, the doctor's questions to Michelle are quite vague (see lines 18 and 20); however, they do not just constitute "small talk," nor do they only serve to pass the time as the doctor analyzes Michelle's medical situation. Whether or not the doctor is actually even remotely curious about Michelle as a student, the critical part is that she opts to acknowledge that part of Michelle as salient (at least to Michelle) by introducing it. The initiation of talk about Michelle as a student, especially the query about her grade, is interesting given the immediate prior exchange where Michelle presents herself (and is affirmed as) an almost-adult who can competently describe her symptoms. As in Excerpt 8 (which occurs later in their interaction), the doctor makes issues that are not necessary to the medical task of doing the physical examination relevant in the conversation. In so doing, the doctor simultaneously recognizes *both* Michelle's medical concerns—and the concurrent medical examination and tasks—*and* parts of her identity that could have legitimately been left on the periphery.

Excerpt 8:

```
 1   C:   Yeah (.10) Well, so, is your brother still livin with you
 2        all, or is he=
 3   P:   =No, no, he moved in with his girlfriend's parents
 4   C:   [okay]
 5   P:   [unintelligible] Her parents own Skate Land
 6   C:   Riiight. See, I had, yeah, I, in fact, I saw him at Skate
 7        Land. I had taken my little girl to a party there.
 8        Well, [that's good]
 9   P:         [Was it the other night?]
10   C:   Noo, it's been a couple of months.
11        [Yeah, it's been a month.]
12   P:   [Cause they had a party] the other night.
13   C:   really?
14   P:   yeah
15   C:   Weell, that's neat. And so the kids are with him?
16   P:   mmhmm
```

17	C:	Well, that's good. I know that was kinda hard on you
18		having them there.
19	P:	I know. It drove me crazy.
20	C:	(laughs) (.3) Are you allergic to any antibiotics,
21		Michelle?
22	P:	mmm mmm The only thing my mom don't like me takin is
23		aspirin.
24	C:	Yeeah. Okay. (.2) Well, let's go with Bactrin. It's a
25		good antibiotic. You can get it in generic, so it's
26		not too expensive, and it's real good for sinuses.
27		(.4) And we'll just take you up to (unintelligible) for
28		fourteen days. (.20) So is it just you and your mom at
29		home now?

Particularly in lines 17 and 18, the doctor demonstrates interest in and concern for Michelle as more than just someone with a sinus infection. Referring to Michelle's disclosures that nieces and nephews (who had been living with Michelle and her mother and brother) moved in with their dad and his girlfriend's family, the doctor offered an assessment of that change by saying, "Well, that's good. I know that was kinda hard on you having them there." Jones explained that such utterances constitute social support and work to "display analysis of ongoing talk by conveying an evaluation of good/bad, right/wrong, true/false, etc. of an assessable" (1994, p. 4; see also Jones, in press).

Michelle affirmed the assessment by responding, "I know. It [having the kids in the house] drove me crazy." The doctor's subsequent laughter attended to the potential laughable ("it drove me crazy"). The assessment and the shared laughter in particular facilitated both facework and identification. The doctor expressed empathy for Michelle's situation while reflexively providing an interactional opportunity for Michelle to provide her own commentary on the family situation. The doctor, not Michelle, first referred to having the kids in the house as "hard"; thus, the doctor would likely not chastise Michelle for a similar observation. By sharing in this "backstage-off-the-record" type of behavior (see Goffman, 1959), the two co-achieved a moment of "connectedness," a "just-between-us-ness," and in so doing, they temporally hesitated on a sliver of common ground.

This snippet of conversation permits the caregiver and patient to interactionally drift amidst the waves of Michelle's multiplicity of identities—including aunt, sister, daughter, near-adult (not "just a kid" so that she may comment on other "kids"). None of those identities disappear, however, as the tide of the conversation gently bobs further to medical tasks once more (see line 20).

In fact, Michelle includes a reference to her mother in response to the doctor's question about allergies. Despite that reference, the doctor does not dwell on Michelle as a daughter, or even a child who defers to her mother's preferences with regard to medication. Instead, the doctor acknowledges that preference and then talks to Michelle about the benefits of the drug that she is being prescribed—efficiency and cost, thus giving credence to Michelle's multidimensional self (child, daughter, consumer, participant, even partner).

In Michelle's case, the doctor's recognition of her multiplicity of identities may not stem directly from the medical tasks at hand. However, the lack of strict medical necessity for this conversation does not undercut its significance to the interactants, especially the patient. This doctor's willingness to talk to her in terms of her multiplicity, her complexity, lays a pivotal foundation for future interactions, for a partnership dynamic. This interaction demonstrates mutual trust, respect, and comradery; it encompasses the nurturing of the patient's identities beyond (but always including) her medical problem.

In Excerpts 9, 10 and 11, the female doctor talks further with Susan, the female patient who wanted the doctor to prescribe Annaprox for pain from menstrual cramps. In these excerpts, the doctor and Susan share information as well as emphasize commonalities that extend beyond the door of the examining room. This portion of their conversation takes place about 5 minutes after the segment that was described in Excerpt 3.

Excerpt 9:

```
103   C:   What kind of work do you do?=
104   P:   =I teach at the university.=
105   C:   =Oh, you do?=
106   P:   =yeah=
107   C:   =Oh great what field?
108   P:   archaeology=
109   C:   =Oh, how interesting. I've always thought that'd be a
110        fascinating [area]
111   P:              [It is.] It's great; it's great.=
112   C:   =So, you like it=
113   P:   =I do, uh=
114   C:   That's wonderful=
115   P:   =yeah
```

In Excerpt 9, the female doctor and Susan reciprocally disclose information and mutually affirm aspects of each other. Susan responds to the doctor's question about her occupation by noting that she teaches "at the university"—making it clear that she "teaches" as opposed to doing some other sort of work. Interestingly, Susan refers only to "the university" as her place of employment, thus, taking for granted that the doctor will know which university; the city in which this interaction occurs has several universities, colleges, and community colleges within driving distance, yet she says "the" university. By not asking Susan to elaborate, the doctor implies that they share understanding of which university, demonstrates interest by commenting that that is "great," and displays her own knowledge about academia by inquiring "what field" (line 107). After discovering that Susan works in archaeology, the doctor compliments her by stressing "how interesting. I've always thought that'd be a fascinating area" (lines 109–110). Susan concurs the doctor's description of her field in line 111 by saying "it's great," and the doctor pursues the topic once more by commenting "so you like it."

Through her affirming statements (see lines 109–110 and 114), the doctor goes beyond simply asking Susan about her work. She shows interest in archaeology and in Susan's happiness in that area. Although the doctor is an expert in medicine, she talks admiringly about Susan's involvement in a field that is very different from her own, giving credence to Susan's professional status as a professor in that field, thus acknowledging that fragment of Susan's life. Notably, the doctor could have moved to her next question after line 104. The choice not to do so suggests genuine interest, not the mere completion of an intake form. In Excerpt 10, the doctor continues her conversation with Susan.

Excerpt 10:

116	C:	Good, do you have any children?
117	P:	We have one. He's eight.
118	C:	Ohh, great
119	P:	Great age
120	C:	Oh, it is, isn't it? My little girl's gonna be eight in
121		a few weeks.
122	P:	What school does she go to?
123	C:	uh, Jackson=
124	P:	=Jackson okay we go to Lincoln=
125	C:	=to Lincoln=
126	P:	=yeah=
127	C:	=okay yeah, that's neat=
128	P:	=but they're all good schools. I don't know that any
129		[(unintelligible)]
130	C:	[Yeah, we've been real happy]=
131	P:	=yeah=
132	C:	=We've been real happy here. Well, um, is your husband
133		also a professor?=

After "good," the doctor integrates yet another part of Susan into the conversation—the "mom" to add to the consumer, the concerned patient, the pain sufferer, the woman, the professional, the faculty member, the archaeologist. In Excerpt 9, the doctor takes a "one-downish" position, admiring her patient's participation in a field that she finds intriguing. In Excerpt 10, the doctor and Susan engage in a more symmetrical interaction, highlighting the "mom" aspect of their busy lives as working mothers and professionals.

Here again, the taken-for-granted reifies their reciprocally co-produced individual and relational identities. When the doctor discloses that her daughter will be "8 in a few weeks" (lines 120–121), Susan asks which school the daughter attends, taking for granted that the question is appropriate and salient. As fellow moms, such a question becomes quite legitimate. Mothers on playgrounds routinely ask the same question of strangers with children. However, it works here to downplay—not get rid of—other dynamics that are simultaneously being enacted (i.e., the doctor–patient implied hierarchy–power differential), especially because the patient asks the question. For this fraction in time, they are moms of kids in school, not just doctor and patient facing similar concerns and struggles amidst all of their other individual and relational identities.

Such a question also serves to bring in underlying issues of social status and degree of wealth. School district assignments depend on place of residence; place of residence implies financial stature. For the "professor" to ask the "doctor," the answer may not be face-threatening or intimidating for either; for the "patient" to ask the "doctor," it could be more awkward and potentially treated as "inappropriate" or "too personal." Susan displays her comfort with disclosing her son's school as well as her lay assumption that the doctor—someone of presumably similar socioeconomic status—would not be disturbed about sharing such information either. She also reflexively positions herself in light of even more aspects of herself (i.e., active mom who knows about the quality of schools, affluent, equal).

After Susan's assessment that "they're all good schools" (line 128), the doctor does not give a direct response except to say that "we've been real happy here" (lines 130 and 132). The doctor's repetition of this reaction (which includes the word "we") and a slight disfluency permits her to ask more about the patient's "we."

Excerpt 11:

```
132   C:   =We've been real happy here. Well, um, is your husband
133        also a professor?=
134   P:   =Yes, and he's going to be coming to YOUR husband=
135   C:   =oh yeah we have a lot of that
136   P:   [Yeah] (laughs)
```

137   C: [Isn't that nice?]
138   P: Yeah I prefer to see a woman; he doesn't care=
139   C: =riight=
140   P: =uhm, yeah, he also teaches in the archaeology department=
141   C: =oh really?=
142   P: =so=
143   C: =oh, that's neat
144   P: Yeaahh, it has its moments=
145   C: =I bet=
146   P: =It's sort of probably like the two of you=
147   C: =riight=
148   P: working together
149   C: [Overall, it's worth it]
150   P: [something's (unintelligible)]
151   C: yeah=
152   P: =yeah, we like it too, but there are times when=
153   C: =yeah=
154   P: =hmm=
155   C: =makes it a little tricky=
156   P: =yeah=
157   C: yeah well okay have you ever had any uh surgeries?

Given that Susan is a married professional, the doctor guesses that Susan's husband might be a professor as well, a guess that makes more sense when we learn that the doctor is also married to another doctor in the same practice. As Susan reveals that her husband intends to visit with the doctor's husband, the interwoven, overlapping nature of their individual and relational identities becomes more evident. All of those identities lurk within their emergent relationship; all are simultaneously salient. While, at one moment, they laugh about the wife visiting the wife and the husband visiting the husband (lines 134–139), in the next they talk about the pros and cons of working with a spouse, occasionally even finishing the other's thought. For example, Susan observes "there are times when" (line 152), and the doctor finishes with "makes it a little tricky" (line 155). A turn at talk later, the doctor inquires about Susan's surgical history (line 157).

Susan's interaction with the doctor in Excerpts 3, 9, 10, and 11 exemplifies a postmodern relationship with a health caregiver. They co-accomplished a multifaceted relational dynamic as they explored and indicated their commonalities, enabling them to achieve identification and facework with regard to a number of individual and relational identities. The doctor provided Susan with a peek at the doctor's multiple selves and afforded Susan an opportunity to present herself as multidimensional and complex. Susan shared in that exchange by asserting herself and her own ideas. They laid a solid foundation for a partnership dynamic in which both of these diverse individuals may play an active part and in which medical decisions may be reached in light of the scattered nature of this patient's life.

In Excerpt 12, the female doctor interacts with "Annie," a female college student. This excerpt exemplifies how the recognition of a multiplicity of patient identities can be more directly tied to medical task interactions. In this case, the doctor invites discussion about the applicability of a certain drug for the student's lifestyle.

Excerpt 12:

```
 1   C:   Um, the typical dosage that they suggest for it is 200
 2        milligrams five times a day. Now that's kind of a pain.
 3        You can also get it in 800 milligrams that's really used
 4        more for genital herpes=
 5   P:   =mm hmm
 6   C:   We just happened to have some of the 800 milligrams at home
 7        from the drug rep sent us, so I took that for this, and
 8        I, I don't know if I should even be telling you this
 9        because a typical dose is 200 five times a day, but I
10        took that, I took one of those, and it just knocked it
11        out=
12   P:   =Really?
13   C:   Yeah, and I just know for a busy college student it might
14        be hard to take [something five times a day]
15   P:                   [five times a day]
16   C:   So, if you want, we can try the 800=
17   P:   =That would be great because=
18   C:   =That might be easier, lemme because then you would take it
19        less often=
20   P:   =mm hmm=
21   C:   =you know, maybe=
22   P:   =well=
23   C:   =once to twice a day=
24   P:   =My sleeping schedule's so strange it's hard for me to take
25        it something three times a day [unintelligible]
26   C:                                  [right] right=
27   P:   =right=
28   C:   =yeah=
29   P:   =yeah=
30   C:   =Okay, well, let me getcha a prescription for that. It
31        helps. Um, at least, it sure cuts down on, you know, the
32        root of it and everything, so yeah. If you know that
```

33		something's coming up that you just can't have a fever
34		blister for=
35	P:	=yeah=
36	C:	=you can always take a few, you know, you can take one for
37		a couple days to make sure, if you're getting your
38		pictures done [or something like that]
39	P:	[Well, it's real] um I get em I know from
40		stress, but if I'm out in the sun, they're all on my
41		face. So it's kinda nice if I get sunburned=
42	C:	=riight=
43	P:	=then I know I I it's just=
44	C:	=you're gonna uh=
45	P:	I know if I get sunburned I'm gonna get one=
46	C:	=You're gonna get one. Riight yeah yeah=
47	P:	=so=
48	C:	=Yeah, yeah, you can take those, and in that instance, they
49		should prevent it, and I can't promise a hundred percent=
50	P:	=oh I know=
51	C:	=but it will [[Tape cuts off]]

In Excerpt 12, the doctor observes that the "typical dose" requires patients to take the drug "five times a day" (line 2). She could have chosen to write the prescription in light of the usual dosage, sent Annie on her way, and moved on to her next patient. Instead, she opts to concede that the required frequency of consumption is "kind of a pain" (line 2) and proceeds to reveal that the drug does come in higher doses. The doctor discloses this information as "between you and me" by confessing that "I don't know if I should even be telling you this" (line 8) and then by sharing her own account of taking one pill that "knocked it out" (lines 10 and 11).

Notably, Annie does not demand this "super pill." She does not say "that's what I want" or "that would work best for me." Annie might have done so later in the conversation; however, the doctor makes this drug especially relevant for the patient in lines 13 and 14. Although not maintaining that this strength of medication is medically necessary for this particular patient, the doctor suggests that this dosage might be appropriate for the patient because of Annie's lifestyle as a "busy college student" (line 13). Only then does Annie start to advance her own position about the inconvenience of the "5 times a day" (line 15).

This demonstration of understanding about the patient by the doctor works in a number of ways to facilitate the relational activities of facework and identification and a multiplicity of patient identities as well as to accommodate medical goals. First, the doctor treats the patient as multifaceted. Annie wants to clear up her blisters, but she must do so amidst the rest of her scattered life. Her life does not simply revolve around the removal of blisters, no matter how much she might want them to be gone. The doctor overtly specifies the paradox for Annie—she wants to get rid of the blisters, but time restrictions could prevent her from doing so if she receives the typical dosage. Through the doctor's reference to the patient as a "busy college student" and as someone who has still more events in her life (such as "getting your pictures done"), the doctor implicitly acknowledges the patient as more than someone who wants to resolve a health care concern.

Second, the sharing of a confidence (line 8) and the sensitivity to what college life involves enables the doctor to initiate a common ground with her patient. The collaborative co-achievement of identification ensues as Annie agrees with the doctor's assertion that pills might be hard to take "five times a day." In fact, after Annie mentions her strange sleep schedule, the doctor and Annie continue to co-affirm that both agree (see lines 26–30), resulting in the doctor's offer to "getcha a prescription for that."

Third, this process of identification facilitates, and is co-achieved through, artful attention to the patient as a multifaceted person. The sculpting of this common ground does not constitute fence-building, separating selves on one side or another (caregiver vs. patient, student vs. patient, etc.). In fact, the doctor even refers to her own status as a patient who took the 800 milligram version of the pill (lines 8–11). Thus, through their identification, they reflexively engage in facework—advancing and reaffirming a plethora of identities that are intertangled.

In terms of both facework and identification, it is important to note what did not occur but which could have been said. The doctor could have dispensed the typical dosage without giving other options. The doctor could have teased Annie by mentioning the other option but refusing to prescribe it. Annie could have protested the five times a day requirement of the typical dosage, and the doctor could have imposed a false hierarchy: Choose which matters more—no blisters or less inconvenience. Even if the super pill was not an option, even if Annie's condition required medication that would be awkward or uncomfortable, the doctor's realization of the both–and preference (and paradox) can help that doctor to discuss any available alternatives with Annie, to help Annie to make good choices, not necessarily perfect ones. In this case, the doctor could and did talk with Annie about viable options, and in so doing, reflexively facilitated facework and identification.

Fourth, the partnership-like orientation of this encounter, the team-like decision-making process wherein the multifaceted patient is appreciated and wherein that patient collaborates on decisions, enhances medical goals. Although we discuss the relationship between relational activities and medical goals in Chapter 5 in much more depth, we want to observe here in this exemplar that the relational activities of facework and identification and the conversational initiative that the caregiver took in raising the complicated nature of the patient's life combine to result in a workable recommendation for the patient and her treatment. Given what the doctor assumes and then learns during the encounter, that patient would not have been able to take the drug as prescribed in the typical dosage. Likely, that drug would not have been effective; the patient would have been frustrated, and the problem would have been left unresolved. As this section has stressed, references to the multiplicity of patient identities is consequential and is imperative for the co-production of a partnership-like dynamic for caregivers and patients.

Multiplicity of Caregiver Identities.   In Excerpt 12, the doctor implies an appreciation of the life of a college student. As a medical doctor, she certainly must have gone to college somewhere, experiencing the time pressures, the diversity of activities and obligations. The doctor's description of Annie's lived reality, which rings true to that patient, provides a peek at a part of herself that becomes salient in her effort to reach out to the patient. More directly, the doctor discloses a specific instance as a patient when she took the 800 milligram version of the drug that she wants to prescribe for her patient. Again, the doctor parts the curtains of her own complicated self, enabling the patient to catch glimpses of fragments of the person who encompasses more than just the "doctor" title.

As this portion of the chapter exemplifies further, personal disclosures by caregivers help to alleviate the imbalance of information exchange between caregivers and patients. Additionally, as in many of the excerpts reviewed thus far, personal disclosures reveal bits of the caregivers beyond their handling of medical tasks, and, reflexively and simultaneously, they contribute to the co-achievement of facework and identification.

Excerpt 13:

1	C:	Yeah, yeah, well, sounds like if you've gotta go to work
2		you just can't do it=
3	P:	=No, I can't
4	C:	oh bless your heart. Th-you know, this happened to me
5		right after I had my last baby, this low back pain, and
6		I never, it gives me such a new appreciation for how
7		patients [feel (laugh)]
8	P:	[shares laughter]
9	C:	Because it, I mean, it's just horrible.
10	P:	If you've never had it before. I never had=
11	C:	=Right. You never understand how bad it is=
12	P:	=No, I'd never had it, and I was like, wow! okay!
13	C:	=No, I finally, my mom worked on it for one one, and I
14		mean like for twenty minutes, constantly, and it hurt
15		so bad=

```
16   P:   =oh sure=
17   C:   =and the next day it was tender but then it went away even
18        because that muscle spasm she had worked all away=
19   P:   =Why? Does it work and work and work?
20   C:   I would have him keep working on it, you know, I sure
21        would
22   P:   =okay=
23   C:   But, um, but, just in case, I think it's a good idea to
24        have the physical therapy back up=
25   P:   =Oh, I think so too
```

In Excerpt 13, the female doctor responds to her patient's ("Dianne") complaint about postpartum lower back pain. In so doing, she shares her own experience as a mother, as a patient, as a person in pain, as a person who can truly understand because of that time and discomfort after childbirth. However, she does so in a way that we can see the blend, the overlap, the both–and-ness of her multiplicity of identities. The doctor empathizes with Dianne as a "new mom," but she does so by still also marking herself as a doctor.

In lines 4 through 7, the doctor explains that "this happened to me right after I had my last baby, this low back pain, and I never, it gives me such a new appreciation for how patients feel." The doctor reveals that she had more than one child; she had a "last baby," implying that there were more before that one. However, she also notes that she had never suffered the pain before that child. Hence, her ability to deeply understand the pain of others—patients—who had postpartum lower back pain changed after the birth of that last child; she gained "such a new appreciation," and she specifies that that "appreciation" was for "patients," not just other moms. After Dianne shares her laughter in line 8, the doctor emphasizes that "it's just horrible," and she reiterates in line 11 that others who have not felt such pain could "never understand how bad it is" and in lines 14 and 15 that "it hurt so bad."

In so doing, the doctor displays herself as someone who *can* legitimately understand, someone who truly "feels her pain." This identification between the doctor and Dianne lays the groundwork for Dianne to heed the doctor's opinion—after all, she does comprehend the agonizing pain; she has been there before. Such a disclosure also permits Dianne to avoid embarrassment about talking about her pain; the doctor agrees that the hurt is real and that the hurt is significant. Through this acknowledgment, the doctor treats Dianne's concern as viable, instead of discarding it as "silly" or "part of the process."

Furthermore, she affirms Dianne's effort to resolve the discomfort. Dianne's husband had been rubbing her back, and the doctor encourages

Dianne to have him continue to do so. In fact, doctor provides Dianne with yet another glimpse of the doctor as multidimensional—the doctor and the patient, the mom and the daughter, the person who helps reduce pain and the person who has suffered from it.

In lines 13 through 15, the doctor reveals that her mom worked on her back in an effort to resolve the pain, just as Dianne's husband was trying to help her. The doctor explains that "it [the pain] went away," just as Dianne's pain could end because of her husband's efforts. However, despite the success of her own lay treatment of her back, the doctor draws Dianne's attention back to the assistance that can be found in the medical community by noting in line 23 through 24 that "just in case, I think it's a good idea to have the physical therapy back up." Dianne readily agrees.

Once again, the doctor demonstrates an appreciation for Dianne's lived reality by describing that reality in a way that resonates for the patient and, in this case, by talking about her own experiences. She carves a distinction between people who could really understand that pain and those who could not as she admitted her own ability to really "get it" before her own suffering (as opposed to her implied inability to truly understand prior to that experience.)

For example, in Excerpt 14, the same doctor interacts with another patient ("Barb") while conducting a pelvic examination. Barb notes that the perineum seems tight since her last episiotomy, and the doctor recounts her own experience.

Excerpt 14:

```
1    P:    It just seems a little tight since then. Of course, my
2          husband doesn't mind.
3    C:    Men make jokes about that. I remember when Dr. ____
4          delivered me. Of course, my husband was just standing
5          right there, and he said, "Well, well, just sew her up a
6          little more." I thought, "I don't need that right now.
7          I just had a baby."
```

Taking a modernist orientation, the doctor presents herself as one who, like the patient, can understand (as opposed to others who cannot). In Excerpt 14, the two relate because of a common medical procedure as well as a similar relational sidebar of that procedure—husbands not "getting" that such procedures hurt and add to distress. As in Excerpt 13, the doctor and Barb facilitate disclosure as women, wives, mothers, and patients.

Especially in these two exemplars, we wonder if such identification and facework would be possible (or even attempted) if the doctor had been male. We tend to think not—the casual references to postpartum back pain and episiotomies would likely not occur in mixed company in Western culture. Furthermore, given the nature of the doctor and patient comments—particularly in Excerpt 14, male caregivers may not be viewed or treated as receptive or understanding listeners for such complaints.

Through intimate personal disclosures, this doctor provides her patients with a glance at the multiplicity of her selves, with, we believe, relational and medical consequences. By telling her stories, she lets her patients in on the complexity of her life and her self. She becomes more than a doctor while remaining a doctor; she arises as "one of us" as opposed to "one of them" (one who has gone through similar trials, not someone who has not) while simultaneously remaining still a health caregiver with enough distance on the situation and abundant professional expertise to offer assistance—thus, paradoxically, not "just" one of "us."

Furthermore, references to the doctor's multiplicity of identities reflexively facilitated particular emergent relational identities. In Excerpts 13 and 14, the female doctor and her patients collaboratively co-achieve the connectedness, the sharedness, of postpartum experiences. Through that bond, they affirmed each other's experiences as well as their emergent individual and relational identities, fellow women, fellow mothers, fellow pain endurers, caregiver–patient, partners in pain, partners in triumph over pain.

The attention to both caregivers and patients as complex and multifaceted underlies their collaborative ability to co-produce a relational dynamic that embraces—not excludes—a multiplicity of relational identities—who they are together. Notably, the emergent discussions between caregivers and patients works reflexively and rhetorically to reinforce their multiplicity of respective identities, to facilitate facework and identification, and to lay a foundation for a partnership between multidimensional people.

Multiplicity of Identities and Time

Throughout this chapter, we have pointed to numerous examples where multiple relational and individual identities emerge and become part of the interaction between caregivers and patients. With the exception of Susan's talk with the doctor during an initial visit, most of these recognitions of the participants as complex emerged in the midst of other medical task-specific activities. Although the caregivers who participated in our various studies may have spent slightly more time with their patients than the norm, we contend that they facilitated the co-accomplishment of relational activities and goals while, at the same time, keeping the encounter "on track" for completion in an expedient period of time. They did so by carefully offering metacommunicative cues that they needed to highlight another aspect of their relational dynamic, not to ignore or eliminate other aspects.

In most cases, initiations of possible interactional framing came from caregivers, thus reflexively perpetuating their authority to alter the focus of the conversation (see also work by Frankel, 1990; Heath, 1986; Modaff, 1995). In many ways, interactional framing in the postmodern era resembles televisions with on-screen co-viewing of more than one channel. The television picture emphasizes one channel by presenting that picture as larger than the rest; however, a few select others stay on the screen albeit in smaller proportions; even more channels continue broadcasting and may be tapped with the flick of a finger on a remote control, thus becoming one of the highlighted images as opposed to underlying ones. In the case of health care encounters, caregivers tend to "hog" the remote more than their patients, thus, again, implying that caregivers and patients both can "channel surf" but that caregivers may strike the previous channel button at will, returning the participants once again to the medical channel and to their medical tasks. Patients rarely fight for control of the remote nor dispute abrupt channel changes; in this regard, they behave and are treated as well-mannered visitors in their doctor's den.

In our data sets, caregivers marked their preferences for re-emphasizing the medical nature of the visit through some combination of the use of "okay" as well as disfluencies and pauses. Notably, this finding is quite consistent with the work of other scholars of interaction in the health care context (see Beach, 1995; Drew & Heritage, 1992; Frankel, 1990; Markova & Foppa, 1991; Modaff, 1995). As these scholars observed, the caregiver initiation of "okay" and a subsequent change in topic perpetuates the asymmetry of the encounter and potentially works to end discussion on an issue of concern to the patient before the patient indicates a preference to do so. Hence, the paradox for the caregiver: She needs to return to the medical business in order to complete the encounter in a timely manner; however, to do so, she might suggest that she is no longer interested in that previous aspect of the conversation (and of the patient's identity and goals) and that it is no longer relevant. Yet, because all fragments of their respective and mutual identities impact each other, nothing can just be written off as "irrelevant." The murky paradox forces transitional awkwardness, especially if a relational problem in another aspect of their dynamic clearly remains unresolved.

For example, in the case of the nurse practitioner's interaction with Nancy (Excerpt 4), the nurse practitioner's potential extention of the laughable is not reciprocated, and the nurse practitioner responds with several seconds of disfluency before recovering (see lines 21–23). However, in Excerpt 6, the nurse practitioner and Melissa share laughter after the pelvic examination and before moving on to some other part of the examination. In that between portion of the encounter, Melissa offers a potential laughable in response to the just-finished examination following a time of silence. To extend the laughter sequence or to dwell on that bit of humor further would not have made sense. Thus, the "okay" does not work to cut some part of the conversation off.

Overall, "okay" seems to serve in a modernist way to move the conversation rigidly from one topic to another, without considering the inherent overlap of the issues and identities. For example, in Excerpt 7, the doctor notes "that's good" in response to Michelle's answer that she is in the ninth grade, pauses, and then says "okay well your lungs sound good" (lines 24–25). Although the necessary re-emphasis of medical business takes place, it does so at the risk of disconfirming the fine relational work that has preceeded it (i.e., "that's nice but now it doesn't matter—let's move on to the important stuff"). Through modernistic separations of systems—the medical system versus the personal system, the intertangling of identities does not get addressed. For a holistic, partnership-like dynamic to emerge, caregivers and patients must find a way continually to revisit and re-orient to the relevance, the importance, of their complex, multifaceted individual and relational identities.

An excellent exemplar of how caregivers and patients may weave their multiplicity of identities throughout the encounter is Excerpt 12, the doctor's interaction with Annie about the blister medication. The doctor and Annie integrate a multiplicity of identities into that exchange as well as to mark the medical salience of those identities. If references to aspects of the interactants become treated as "just asides," both caregivers and patients interactionally undermine their importance in the ever-evolving relational dynamic; they cannot be cast aside as "outside influences" that really have no bearing on the system at hand.

A REVIEW

In this chapter, we have discussed the consequential and reflexive nature of relational and conversational activities. Although previously treated as modernist conceptions, we re-visit work on facework, identification, and interactional framing and illustrate their importance in postmodern discussions of interpersonal relationships, particularly in the health care context. Through the excerpts that we include in this chapter, we demonstrate how health caregivers and patients may engage in conversational activities that work reflexively to facilitate facework, identification, and interactional framing. Further, we note the reflexive implications for those relational activities on the co-accomplishment of a partnership dynamic.

This chapter lays the groundwork for the next two chapters on the co-achievement of educational and medical goals. We contend that it is through the reflexivity of conversational and relational activities that those goals may be expediently and efficiently co-accomplished by caregivers and patients. Notably, in this chapter, we primarily chose exemplars of interaction that demonstrate, for the most part, how these relational activities can be achieved, reserving examples in which the interactants do not attend to facework and identification as well for the next two chapters. It is in those chapters that we hope to indicate the consequentiality and reflexivity of relational goals for how patient education as well as medical tasks occur during health care encounters.

The Co-Accomplishment of Educational Goals

"Leslie," a nurse on the surgical floor of a midsized, midwestern hospital, had just started her rounds when she met "Mrs. Applebee." As part of my ethnographic research at the hospital, I followed Leslie into the double-occupancy hospital room, past the empty first bed, and over to the bed by the window. Leslie picked up Mrs. Applebee's chart from the end of the bed, quickly scanned it, and then looked at the frail elderly woman in the bed—Mrs. Applebee. Mrs. Applebee smiled at both of us, her alert eyes beaming from behind the rims of her glasses. "My," she said, "visitors so soon."

Leslie glanced at me and then met Mrs. Applebee's gaze and returned her smile. "Hello, Mrs. Applebee. I see that you've had quite the morning," Leslie said. Mrs. Applebee shook her head and sighed. "I can't believe my luck. One moment I'm fine, and the next minute, I'm flat on my back wondering how on earth I'm going to phone for help," Mrs. Applebee said. "So, you took a fall this morning?" Leslie asked. "Mm hmm," Mrs. Applebee answered, "right there in my kitchen. I'd never broken a bone in my body. Eighty-three years old, never a one."

However, as Leslie continued her conversation with Mrs. Applebee, she learned that Mrs. Applebee had had her share of health problems over the years. None of those problems had been life-threatening, but the arthritis and osteoporosis made movement increasingly painful.

Leslie also discovered that Mrs. Applebee lived alone in the two-story house that she had called home with Mr. Applebee for 53 years; her husband had died 2 years earlier. Leslie inquired about Mrs. Applebee's children, and Mrs. Applebee told us that her two "super" and "considerate" children now lived in other states with "great careers" and "families of their own." Only a niece still resided near her. According to Mrs. Applebee, the niece "checks in on me every week or so." When asked about nearby friends or neighbors, Mrs. Applebee explained that many of her long-time friends and neighbors had either died or moved away to "some old folks' home." However, Mrs. Applebee hastened to add that "I don't get lonely because my kitty keeps me company." Mrs. Applebee also proudly commented that she "gets around pretty well," doing her own shopping, her own driving, and even her own yard work until this last year "when my back got too stiff."

Leslie spent about 20 minutes with Mrs. Applebee, hearing her stories about her illnesses and her previous medical experiences, listening to her descriptions of her husband, niece, and cat. Finally, Leslie asked, "Mrs. Applebee, do you know why you were admitted to the hospital?" "Yes," Mrs. Applebee replied quietly, "I broke my hip." Leslie looked at this proud, independent woman and said, "That's right. You have been scheduled for surgery for tomorrow morning." Leslie paused for a few moments and then continued, "Mrs. Applebee, what kind of arrangements would you like to make for after the surgery?" Mrs. Applebee's forehead creased, and a puzzled look came upon her face. "Why, I'll go home, of course."

With Mrs. Applebee's health history and the impending hip operation, Leslie knew that Mrs. Applebee likely would not return to her two-story home of 53 years for a long, long time, if ever, especially because she lacked close family members or neighbors to assist her. Leslie tried to explain, "Mrs. Applebee, it will be hard for you to walk after the surgery. I'm afraid that you'll need someone to help you. Most people who have this kind of surgery have to stay in some long-term care facility during their recovery period. I see that you do have insurance so you won't have to worry about—" Mrs. Applebee interrupted her, appearing upset for the first time in the health care encounter, "but my kitty, what about my kitty? I'm sure that she'll be concerned about me, and now that I think about it, I'm not sure that those emergency people even made sure that she was in the house when they carried me out. I had to go on a stretcher, you know."

When we left Mrs. Applebee's room later, I felt drained and helpless. This independent yet frail woman had no one to care for her, no one to call to check on her cat or on the money from her social security check that she had just cashed, put in her "safe" place, and needed to take to the bank. I found myself wanting to volunteer to go to her house, to lock things up, to confirm that her "kitty" had food and water. I could not imagine lying in her place, alone in a hospital bed, wanting to turn back the clock to the hour before the fall, craving the simple freedom that mobility brings, desiring the comfort of my cat and my house. I also could not conceptualize what it must have been like for her to hear the news that she might not be able to experience that freedom, to touch her cat, to walk into her house "for a long, long time."

"Is this hard for you?" I asked Leslie as we walked down the hall to the next patient's room. She thought for a moment and then said, "No, I guess that I've accepted that there is a whole lot that I can't change. I can't change the fact that that woman is alone. I can't save everyone's cat. So, I focus on what I can do." "What's that?" I asked. She slowed down and turned to me. "I guess that I can let them know what's coming or what might come so that they can do the best that they can with their situations," Leslie said.

In the emotion of the moment, I thought that her reaction was somewhat cold. I wondered how she could not help but feel for that woman, to want to reach out to her, to want to help Mrs. Applebee find someone to take care of her and her cat. As I visited with more health care professionals during my ethnographic work, however, I learned that many of their ways of reaching out to and caring for patients resemble the descriptions of caregivers that Montgomery offered in her 1993 book. The approach of those caregivers fits with the words of the "Serenity Prayer" from Alcoholics Anoymous: "God grant me the Serenity to Accept the things I cannot change, Courage to change the things I can and the Wisdom to know the difference."

Caregivers *can* strive to give the best medical care possible; they *can* attempt to provide that care in terms of the multiplicity of identities that inhabit sometimes delicate and broken bodies. Caregivers who want to nurture an interactional environment wherein patients become partners in their health care *can* enable them to sort through options and to make good decisions by fostering the process of interactive patient education (see also Ragan, Beck, & White, 1995). In the case of Leslie and Mrs. Applebee, the nurse could not alter the facts that the patient fell, that she broke her hip, that she was alone, that she faced a new, less independent life at least during the recovery process. However, Leslie could (and did) discuss alternatives with Mrs. Applebee so that Mrs. Applebee could make informed, intelligent choices before anesthesia and pain medications impaired her ability to do so.

As we observed in Chapter 1, silence has been a pervasive problem in health care for women, patients not knowing how or what to ask, caregivers not knowing what or how to share. Leslie could have opted to remain silent, to prepare Mrs. Applebee physically for the surgery, and to let others decide where Mrs. Applebee should be sent for long-term care and how her affairs would be handled. Instead, Leslie took the lead by providing information and alternatives in what Haggard (1989) referred to as "that golden moment" when the patient needs answers and assistance in understanding her situation.

A number of scholars call for more attention to patient education, especially in terms of formal and informal health education programs in hospitals and outpatient facilities (see, e.g., Bille, 1981; Falvo, 1985; Haggard, 1989; Squyres, 1980, 1985). Although we readily acknowledge the need for structured patient education (particularly in terms of illnesses like diabetes that require patients to perform procedures on themselves and in terms of preventive health practices and new baby care), we suggest that "that golden moment" often comes during interactions between caregivers and patients when education is not necessarily the top priority of either participant. We maintain that educational goals, like relational goals and medical goals, become intertwined and co-accomplished through other simultaneous activities during health care encounters. When either caregivers or patients opt to stay silent and to assume that information will come from other sources, they miss invaluable opportunities to collaborate on conceptions (or misconceptions) about a multitude of topics, potentially influencing and constraining the likelihood that patients will make informed decisions about their health care and wellness (see Bille, 1981; Falvo, 1985; Haggard, 1989).

In this chapter, we examine how caregivers and patients may co-construct interactional opportunities for the co-accomplishment of educational goals. Again, we focus on the issues that the interactants make relevant during the conversation; however, we also note utterances that do not get pursued by the interactants in an attempt to mark missed moments when education could have occurred. As we explore how interactants do (and do not) engage in the process of patient education, we note how relational activities work to facilitate that process—as well as how those activities are reflexively perpetuated through that process.

As Chapter 3 illustrates, the affirmation of both interactants' perspectives can facilitate the recognition—even appreciation—of a multiplicity of individual and relational identities. Through that affirmation, caregivers and patients may co-accomplish facework, identification, and interactional framing, carefully discerning and delineating "who we are" to each other during the encounter and "what may occur here" as they proceed. In this chapter, we suggest that the relational activities of facework, identification, and interactional framing facilitate caregiver and patient co-orientation to the emergent relational dynamic *and* to the sharing of information. Furthermore, we contend that the way in which information exchanges occur works reflexively to impact the interactants' co-achievement of those relational activities. As the following exemplars indicate, even when caregivers and patients fail to accomplish a partnership-like relational dynamic, the very nature of their exchanges of ideas and understandings contributes to (and stems from) their emergent, complex relational co-definition as well as concurrent and reflexive relational activities.

We argue that for a partnership-like relational dynamic to develop, the sharing of knowledge, insight, and understanding must be interactive, participative, respectful, and collaborative. At the very core of any attempt at a partnership-like relational dynamic emanates the idea of mutual respect for their multiplicity of preferred identities and reciprocity of concern for what each brings to, and wants from, the health care encounter (with regard to identities, goals, knowledge, preconceptions, etc.). Just as it is impossible to examine the participants in isolation of each other and their identities in isolation of other identities, it is futile to sequester one set of goals (educational) from another (relational); they are inherently linked together, much like other aspects of the dyadic system. In the following pages, we detail how conversational activities (such as giving and requesting explanations, and initiating and reinforcing participation in the health care process) impact the co-achievement of an interactional environment wherein educational goals may be realized by both caregivers and patients.

GIVING AND RECEIVING OF EXPLANATIONS

As we observe in Chapter 1, caregivers and patients struggle with patient education for a number of reasons. They lack, to varying degrees, a shared language. They may come to their interactions with differing preconceptions about what constitutes "important" and "necessary" facts, beliefs, and ideas to raise and respond to during health care encounters, especially in light of tight time constraints and the plethora of possible topics, sources of information, and complexity of issues. However, even in the mundane taking of a patient history, openings abound for building rapport, for demonstrating respect and appreciation for perspectives and convictions, and for developing a consensus with regard to why some issues should be treated as salient, whereas others are not and of what each interactant means by terms, references, and "facts."

Paradoxically, despite the desire to discuss multiple ideas and concerns simultaneously and despite the reflexivity of language that permits the co-accomplishment of numerous concurrent activities, the nature of conversation limits caregivers and patients with regard to what and how much they can talk about at a single instance of time. Every subject that is relevant to caregivers and patients cannot be made interactionally germane at once. However, those issues do not lose their pertinence to those interactants because they are not constantly vocalized (just as every fragment of identity continues to exist as part of a blurred background while not always coming into focus in the forefront during interactions). Health care participants must struggle with the dilemma of co-determining "a" working understanding of what to discuss and how to co-define circumstances as well as the importance of issues when such singularity undermines the multiplicity of possible understandings, the complexity of intertangled beliefs, desires, and identities. Although the co-achievement of connectedness and shared knowledge between caregivers and patients underlies the notion of patient education, the frustration for caregivers and patients is that such sharedness can never be complete or absolute; it is ever emergent, temporal, and fragmented. As caregivers and patients scramble for solid footing on some elusive steady common ground, they do so amidst the constant quaking and shifting of their worlds, the perpetual disorientation from sundry, swirling, potentially conflicting ways of viewing their realities.

Given the uncertainty and ambiguity of the postmodern era and the multiplicity of identities, goals, and perspectives that each interactant brings to the encounter, the collaborative achievement of explanations is essential to starting a dialogue (instead of caregivers offering just a monologue) about health care concerns. When caregivers overlook opportunities for offering information and when patients postpone probing for answers, the silence can stifle conversations, hinder identification, threaten aspects of identities, and deter a partnership-like orientation to jointly understanding complicated health care and life situations and finding mutually acceptable courses of action.

In this portion of the chapter, we begin by identifying instances of inter-action in which caregivers and patients fail to do a thorough job of requesting or offering more information and explanations. For example, patients may answer some questions in a series of questions by caregivers yet not learn why those questions were posed, why those answers were important, what answers could have been construed as "correct" or "incorrect," and what the implications of the answers are for patient wellness. By not co-facilitating an interactional dynamic wherein differentials in orientations are acknowledged and addressed, caregivers and patients skip past possible patient perspectives and concerns on those topics, perpetuating the gap in understanding between caregivers and patients and contributing to patient frustration and feelings of disconfirmation.

In Excerpts 15, 16, and 17, a caregiver at a Native-American health care facility repeatedly asks "Vicki," a 21-year-old pregnant patient, about her last menstrual cycle. Although Vicki consistently offers the same answer, the nurse, a LPN, fails to acknowledge that Vicki already provided her with that requested response, thus implicitly dismissing Vicki's stance and threatening her self-presentation as someone who knows her own body and history, as someone who can competently report her case, even as someone who tells the truth. The nurse gives no reason for her redundant questions and dem-onstrates little concern for Vicki's participation during this line of questioning.

Excerpt 15:

```
1   C:   When was your last menstrual period?
2   P:   Ah (.) okay (.) I had a normal one in December and then in
3        January I had one but it lasted like two weeks and two
4        days
5   C:   and that was what dates?
6   P:   I think I started on the fourth
```

7	C:	It was abnormal?
8	P:	ah (.) yeah I guess you'd call it abnormal
9	C:	last normal one was in December?
10	P:	um hum
11	C:	December what?
12	P:	ah (.) probably round Christmas time
13	C:	You just had this one right after?
14	P:	okay (.) I think I started around the thirteenth
15	C:	this year?
16	P:	yeah and then=
17	C:	okay (.) last Pap test?

After her clarification question about the period that lasted more than 2 weeks (line 7) and about the "last normal one" occurring in December (line 9), the nurse tries to determine the exact date of the last normal period and then moves to the next topic, asking about Vicki's last Pap smear. Although the nurse expresses a good deal of interest in the specific dates, she does not explain why those dates were important to her or to Vicki. She also gives Vicki reason to believe that her answers have been sufficient by saying "okay" and then inquiring about her "last Pap test" (line 17). Yet, 37 lines later, the nurse initiates the exchange in Excerpt 16, implicitly disregarding what Vicki has just told her about her cycles

Excerpt 16:

54	C:	What is the date of your last period?
55	P:	the one in January?
56	C:	un hun
57	P:	There's no way I could have got pregnant in December
58		since I had that one in January (.1) is there?
59	C:	I don't know (.) Kathleen could probably help you with
60		that (.) figure that out (.) I don't know (laugh)
61	P:	I thought that was for real.
62	C:	okay (.) do you smoke?

In line 55, Vicki responds to the nurse's question by referring her back to the previous discussion. Instead of noting (once more) that "I had one in January," Vicki structures her response as "the one in January?" (line 55), implying that the nurse has prior knowledge of that "one." The nurse acknowledges that prior knowledge with "un hun," not with something like "if that's the last one that you had" (line 56).

In lines 57 through 58, Vicki does not provide the nurse with the specific dates; instead, she asks the nurse a question which suggests that Vicki has a theory about why this information is important—determining the possible date of conception. Vicki asks the nurse if she could have conceived in December, even if she had a period in January. Notably, the nurse does not attend to the assumption that underlies Vicki's question (that the date of conception is the reason that she wants to learn the specific dates) nor to any concerns that Vicki might have regarding her pregnancy because of a possible shift in due dates. Instead, the nurse refers her to Kathleen, the physician's assistant, and laughs briefly.

Vicki does not share the nurse's laughter. She quietly and reflectively notes that "I thought that was for real." Once again, the nurse does not respond to Vicki's apprehensions, help explain what might have happened, or talk to Vicki about the ramifications of the change in due date for the baby. By raising the issue of the dates and then by failing to explain why those dates are salient at this point in the pregnancy, the nurse misses a chance to inform Vicki, to lessen the knowledge differential that separates them, to "bring her up to speed" so that she can participate as a partner in her health care.

However, beyond the missed opportunity, the nurse's choice not to pursue Vicki's expressions of concerns and uncertainty poses potential medical and relational consequences. There may be solid, medical reasons for exploring this topic, reasons that Vicki wants to discuss but that she fears expressing in a more direct manner. For example, Vicki might have taken drugs, consumed alcohol, had intercourse with another partner in December but not in January. Yet, the nurse does not probe deeper into Vicki's perspective to learn about any of these possible lurking issues. The nurse merely says "okay" to Vicki's statement that she "thought it was for real" and then inquires about whether or not she smokes, thus brushing any of Vicki's desires to talk and learn more about this topic aside, implicitly dismissing them rather than encouraging a discussion.

As Smith-Dupre and Beck (1996) and DuPre and Beck (in press) explained, utterances such as "I thought it was for real" can function as "presequences," segments of talk that allude to possible future portions of conversation and that indicate a preference for how the present speaker wishes the next speaker to respond (see Schegloff, 1980). In some of our earlier work, DuPre and Beck (in press) observed that patients may preface bad news for their caregivers by engaging in exaggerated self-disparagement, and Smith-Dupre and Beck (1996) noted that "the introduction of sensitive issues [by patients] is often marked by a preceding string of apologies, disclaimers, abandoned utterances, and contradictory remarks" (p. 80). As DuPre and Beck (in press) contended, especially in the case of turns at talk that begin with some sort of exaggerated self-disparagement (i.e., "I think I mean I'm crazy"), interactants imply what they want the next speaker to address (i.e., "no, you're not crazy").

In any case, presequences entail interactants setting up an implied adjacency pair, with the first pair part involving some issue that the next speaker should respond to with a second pair part. Throughout our data sets, we found that presequences constitute indirect requests by patients to caregivers for information or reassurance and/or for an extension of some aspect of the conversation. However, although interactants in everyday talk routinely seek some sort of repair work or accounting on the part of co-interactants who do not offer the second pair part of adjacency pairs (such as answers to questions; see Sacks, 1992a, 1992b; Schegloff, Jefferson, & Sacks, 1977), patients who advance presequences do not tend to pursue the implied second pair parts (i.e., the desired information or reassurance) from caregivers who fail to provide them. When caregivers do not accept subtle invitations by their patients to speak to their needs, patients treat those invitations as dismissed and denied. Like Vicki, they silently let the subject of the presequence drop instead of pursuing it again indirectly through some meta-comment or laughable (e.g., "Boy, we keep coming back to this one, don't we?") or even more directly (e.g., "How can I figure out what was going on with me in January?" or "Would you explain why the exact date is so important? Is it the baby?")

In line 62, the nurse opts to move to another topic, interactionally closing the door on the dates issue—at least momentarily. In so doing, she slams Vicki's fingers which were left lingering in the entrance way, crushing Vicki's efforts to pry information from the nurse, dashing her attempts to gain reassurance. Perhaps most significantly, however, in the process, the nurse thwarts a chance to understand more about Vicki's medical situation, to attend to a multiplicity of face needs related to Vicki's complex and diverse composite of identities, and to build some common ground of understanding between them. By taking the time to explain why she keeps returning to this topic, why it is important to her and to Vicki, the nurse could attend to Vicki's uncertainties. By taking the time to encourage Vicki's questions and tentatively expressed thoughts, the nurse could demonstrate her concern for Vicki as more than just a patient with medical information to give. Her choice not to do so implicitly disregards those aspects of Vicki and works to separate, not connect, herself from Vicki.

However, the dismissal of those unspoken and unaddressed relational, educational, and perhaps even medical goals becomes even more magnified as the encounter ensues. The disturbing irony of this abrupt and consequential shift to "do you smoke" in line 62 stems from the nurse's decision to revisit the dates issue once more 91 lines later in the conversation. Despite the two exchanges with Vicki about her cycle, especially Vicki's last few utterances in Excerpt 16 about her period in January, the nurse begins Excerpt 17 by claiming ignorance about the unusual nature of the January cycle.

Excerpt 17:

153   C: Your last period in January was normal?
154   P: uh (.) abnormal
155   C: You are certain of that date?
156   P: I am not certain.
157   C: okay (.) You did have one in December though didn't you?
158   P: yes
159   C: and you're twenty-one?

In this portion of their interaction, Vicki starts to show her frustration with the redundancy of the nurse's questions. Vicki responds briefly in line 154 with a slight hesitation and then simply notes that the period in January was "abnormal"; she re-asserts in line 156 "I am not certain" about the date, and she says "yes" to the nurse's inquiry about the period in December. Yet again, without any acknowledgment of the prior conversations, without any additional explanation about the significance or implications of this information, without any displays of concern for the patient and her multiplicity of perspectives or fears, the nurse moves on again with "and you're twenty-one?"

Like so many of the women patients who we referred to in Chapter 1, Vicki refrained from actively seeking information except in Excerpt 16. On the two occasions when Vicki did mark her preference for more details or some sort of reassurance, the nurse did not attempt to give either to Vicki. This series of interactions exemplifies a lack of interactional attention to facework, identification, and patient education. The nurse tightly concealed her hand instead of reaching out to Vicki by noting her perspective and by assisting her in understanding and in sorting through her feelings. Furthermore, even if the nurse did not have specific answers about when Vicki became pregnant, she certainly had some reason for pursuing the dates of the last cycle yet she opted not to share it.

In Excerpt 18, a physician's assistant at the same Native-American health care facility probes to determine whether or not her patient, "Nora," maintains records of her menstrual cycles. Yet, she goes further by describing why such records can be important and by suggesting, not commanding, Nora to note the dates. Although we explore the consequences of such suggestive directives for the co-accomplishment of medical goals in the next chapter, Excerpt 18 offers a good example of the reflexive interplay among relational, educational, and medical goals.

Excerpt 18:

1   C: >do ya< write (.) your periods down (.) >on uh< calendar (.)
2   >at home<?
3   P: u:m no:o (.)

```
 4   C:   oka:y (.) it's really best >if ya< try (.) >to do< that (.)
 5        hhh an make a hhh dal note uh >you know< >monthly habit<
 6        (.)
 7   P:   mmhmm=
 8   C:   =an then hhh when >something like this< happens (.) we have
 9        a< better id[ea]
10   P:               [ha] ha yah=
11   C:   =>ya know< >of what's< going on (.) sometimes we really
12        rely on these pe:riods for (.) hhh a lot of things (.)
13        >not just< pregnancy=
14   P:   =mmhmm=
15   C:   =if you >start having< abnormal ble:eding (.) hhh something
16        (.) >went wrong< with your reproductive sy (.) track (.)
17        hhh we'd need to know=
18   P:   =mmhmm=
19   C:   =so it's real important=
20   P:   =mmhmm=
21   C:   =it's uh >and most women don't remember (.) >I mean< (.)
22        they're so: busy . . .
```

Through her question to Nora in lines 1 through 2, the physician's assistant implies that writing the dates of periods on a calendar is a preferred activity, yet Nora reveals hesitantly that she does not do so in line 3. Hence, the two interactants confront a potentially face-threatening situation as well as one in which patient knowledge, understanding, and future behavior could be impacted by the nature of the discussion.

The physician's assistant does not start with a criticism of Nora's negative response. Instead, she acknowledges the "no:o" and suggests that "it's really best >if ya< try (.) >to do< that." Notably, the physician's assistant phrases her directive as something the patient ought to "try" to do, not has to do or needs to do. In so doing, she gives the patient choice as well as flexibility—she does not give her a condescending lecture (i.e., "You should know to keep those records and you just haven't done it") or an ultimatum ("We can't care for you if you can't give us good information"). (See also related discussion in Chapter 5.)

Significantly, the physician's assistant does not stop with that claim. Instead, she proceeds to offer Nora an explanation, a rationale, for why she should choose to record her periods (lines 8–9, 11–13, 15–17) and concludes by emphasizing that "it's real important." The dilemma for the physician's assistant, however, is that, by giving this explanation to Nora, she implicitly sets up another potentially face-threatening situation—Nora now has unexplained bleeding; they need information yet lack it, and by extension, Nora is to "blame."

The physician's assistant reduces the face implications of her explanation by offering Nora a possible "out" or account (and reflexively, alluding to other aspects of Nora's multifaceted composite of identities—i.e., the woman in the world). The physician's assistant remarks that Nora is not alone; "most women don't remember" (line 21). Furthermore, the physician's assistant implies that those women—like Nora—have a good excuse; "they're so: busy" (line 22). The physician's assistant does not back away from her position that keeping records facilitates the health care process; however, she presents her case by providing information to the patient and by addressing Nora as a multifaceted individual with face needs and preferences.

Ironically, the same physician's assistant at the Native-American health care facility engaged another patient, "Amber," in a less useful discussion of menstrual cycle dates. Although the physician's assistant does say that "it's a good idea [to keep track of cycles] in case anything happens," as in the forenoted excerpts, this caregiver does not explain why, and the patient does not pursue an explanation. Furthermore, the physician's assistant also fails to give credence to Amber's conviction that she remembered the date of her last cycle in Excerpts 19 and 20, thus undercutting Amber's ability to present herself as knowledgeable, competent, and trustworthy. By comparison with Excerpt 18, the following exemplifies the consequentiality of relational activities, particularly with regard to the co-accomplishment of educational goals.

Excerpt 19:

1	C:	okay (.) and your last menstrual period?
2	P:	was September seventeenth
3	C:	okay (.) and you're real positive of that date?
4	P:	well that's yeah
5	C:	okay
6	P:	yeah (.) I remember having a period
7	C:	Do you keep track of your periods?
8	P:	usually I don't but this time I really did
9	C:	okay (.) that's good (.) I always tell them it's a good
10		idea in case anything happens to know when your last
11		menstrual period is (.) you know (.) It's a good date
12		to remember. Did Lora tell you when you were gonna
13		have the baby then?

Amber promptly gives September 17 as the date of her last cycle. The physician's assistant says "okay" and then attempts to assess how certain Amber is about that particular date. Amber prefaces "yeah" with disfluencies in line 4. The physician's assistant responds with "okay," and Amber continues in line 6 by repeating "yeah" and noting "I remember having a period." Thus, although Amber begins by sounding convinced about September 17, she does not reiterate that certainty in her next two turns at talk. Because the date is important and because these health caregivers may have had prior experiences with other women at this clinic who err on reporting dates of cycles, the physician's assistant probes further after these ambiguous responses. The physician's assistant asks, "Do you keep track of your periods?" Such a question enables the physician's assistant to discern whether the date constitutes a viable answer or a guess on the part of the patient (who may offer that "guess" to avoid sounding ignorant or to present herself as someone who has information that the health caregiver obviously expects her to have available).

In this instance, the patient answers by admitting that "usually I don't but this time I really did." The physician's assistant praises her for doing something that she considers to be "a good idea," observing that patients should be aware of that date "in case anything happens" (although not defining what "anything" might be). The physician's assistant then starts to discuss Amber's due date, a logical extension of the conversation from the talk about Amber's last cycle.

The problem occurs several lines later. Although the physician's assistant gives Amber no indication in Excerpt 19 that she doubts her account of the date, in Excerpt 20, she refers to it as less than certain.

Excerpt 20:

92	C:	and today (.) according to your dates (.) if they are
93		correct (.) you are twenty-three and a half weeks
94		pregnant. Now, when you had your cesarean section in
95		Ada (.) did they talk to you about maybe (.) when you
96		got pregnant again (.) about having the baby vaginally
97		or having another c-section (.) or did they talk to you
98		about that at all?
99	P:	They didn't tell me about nothing.
100	C:	(unintelligible) When you have your incision (.) is it
101		straight up and down like this or across like this?
102	P:	no (.) it's up and down (.) straight up and down
103	C:	up and down (.) okay (.) then you want to deliver at
104		Ada?
105	P:	umhum
106	C:	what we'll do is (.) we'll send you down there (.) ah
107		(.) we may have to send you down earlier to get an
108		ultrasound because you're not sure (.) you know (.) for
109		sure (.) if your dates are right (.) we may have to do
110		that (.) but (.) because you've had one c-section
111		doesn't always mean you're going to have another c-
112		section
113	P:	yeah

Despite her implied acceptance of Amber's recollection of the date in Excerpt 19, the physician's assistant suggests that the date may not be accurate in Excerpt 20 (see lines 92, 93, and 108). The physician's assistant makes that assertion in a way that does not even take Amber's claims into account that she did keep track of her period this time and that September 17 is the date. The physician's assistant simply treats those claims as problematic without engaging in any kind of facework to offer Amber a possible "out." Then, in line 108, the physician's assistant disregards Amber's prior stance and implies that *Amber* is the one who is not sure without any interactional indications from Amber that Amber has changed her mind during the course of the conversation.

This kind of disconfirmation hinders the co-accomplishment of facework and identification as well as a partnership-like relational dynamic. If the physician's assistant suggests that she cannot rely on the patient's description of events that involve her own body and if the physician's assistant implies that she can re-write the patient's assertions to fit her own views (and if the patient permits her to engage in those practices without so much as a word or a corrective), then the two cannot treat each other as symmetrical partners who collaboratively—not independently—co-construct the health care encounter, much less co-produce a conducive interactional environment for patient education.

Although the physician's assistant does inform Amber about the possible choice of a vaginal delivery over a repeat c-section, she does not initiate (nor does the patient prompt) efforts to talk completely about the issue of the accuracy of the date nor about the implications of the direction of the incision. The latter might be inferentially linked to the interaction about the repeat c-section, but the lack of discussion about the patient's perspective of the date and the physician's assistant's recasting of that perspective hinders educational and relational goals.

Certainly, the physician's assistant could have re-introduced the issue in a less face-threatening manner (i.e., by saying "for the sake of argument, let's look at how your delivery date could change if your last cycle was September 1 or September 30" or "It's so hard for me to keep track of everything in my life; I can imagine how easy it would be to invert dates"). As she does present it, the physician's assistant denies Amber's view of that particular aspect of reality and likely threatens parts of Amber's identity in the process. Yet, Amber does not contest how the physician's assistant represents her version of the dates issue; she remains silent, implicitly and reflexively reifying the physician's assistant's "right" to depict Amber's level of certainty in this manner. Without some efforts at identification or facework via interactional repair work or some sort of account (see Morris, White, & Itis, 1994, for related work on accounts in conversation), the physician's assistant implicitly positions herself as someone who knows more about

Amber than Amber can legitimately remember. Amber affirms that treatment of her through her silence, perpetuating the asymmetry and intensifying—not diminishing—the knowledge differential on yet another level.

Notably, when Vicki visited later with the same physician's assistant, her health care experience continued in much the same manner as with the nurse who took her medical history, with similar implications for subsequent interactive patient learning. In Excerpt 21, the physician's assistant asks a potentially face-threatening question to Vicki and then brushes aside her answers. In so doing, this physician's assistant at the Native-American health care facility misses a valuable opportunity to build rapport with her patient, to identify with her, to demonstrate consideration for her multiplicity of identities, and most important for the present analysis, to engage Vicki in the process of better understanding her situation.

Excerpt 21:

1	C:	Have you started the pregnancy off overweight?
2	P:	Excuse me?
3	C:	When you started the pregnancy off you were overweight?
4		When you first got pregnant?
5	P:	Now, I've gained an extra 15 pounds probably
6		(unintelligible)
7	C:	okay
8	P:	probably gas
9	C:	right (.) okay (.) How much do you like to weigh? What's
10		a good weight for you?

The physician's assistant begins this series of questions with an almost accusatory comment about Vicki's weight—a very sensitive topic for most women. The physician's assistant's question alludes to some ideal range of weight that Vicki exceeded even before she gained weight with the pregnancy, an "ideal" that Vicki may not necessarily share. Such a question implies a "mistake"; Vicki started the pregnancy in an incorrect manner.

Vicki displays her surprise at the nature of the question by responding with a question instead of a direct answer to the physician's assistant's query. In line 2, Vicki asks, "Excuse me?" The physician's assistant virtually repeats the same question in line 3, insinuating again that Vicki was, indeed, overweight at beginning of her pregnancy. Despite Vicki's initial response, the physician's assistant does not attempt to do any kind of repair or to offer an account for what has been taken as a dispreferred type of question. Notably, as a health care professional who is striving to obtain information, the physician's assistant is not necessarily doing anything "wrong" by engaging in this line of questioning—she has a need to identify possible problems with the pregnancy. The error that mandates a repair involves the lack of regard for the multiplicity of identities (e.g., for the woman who has some degree of pride in her appearance, for the mother-to-be who wants to be taken as "healthy").

After the physician's assistant prompts her again with "when you first got pregnant?" (line 4), Vicki answers, but notably, in terms of what she has gained *since* the beginning of the pregnancy, not with what she weighed *before* the pregnancy. Because she has no way of knowing how the physician's assistant operationalizes "overweight," Vicki could not and did not make an assessment about whether or not her initial weight exceeded some other-defined optimum weight. Interestingly, the physician's assistant does not provide her with that information; she merely acknowledges the response with "okay" in line 7.

At that point, Vicki provides a possible reason for the weight gain—"probably gas"—in line 8. Whereas the "patient" might feel comfortable with just giving "the facts," Vicki constitutes much more than simply a "patient"; that multifaceted individual somehow becomes entangled in a face-threatening situation where she starts to justify why she might have gained what this caregiver perceived as "too much," despite Vicki's own perspective on the weight issue, despite her possible indignance at the tenor of the conversation, and despite her potential lack of understanding about the importance of the issue for her present well-being.

Yet, the physician's assistant does not attend to that face need nor to the understanding or misunderstanding that the patient might have about the weight issue. The closest that the physician's assistant comes to acknowledging the patient's complex perspective occurs through her last two questions in this series to Vicki in lines 9 through 10 ("How much do you like to weigh? What's a good weight for you"). The very positioning of those questions works reflexively to indicate the physician's assistant's prioritizing of viewpoints, and further, her at least initial preference for control over collaboration. In so doing, the physician's assistant negated a chance to make Vicki's perspective the starting point for a dialogue, not an afterthought. By not beginning a conversation with Vicki through these questions, the physician's assistant disregarded opportunities to affirm Vicki as a co-participant, to identify with her on a multitude of levels (including as fellow women), and to explain the implications of the weight issue on some snippet of collaboratively co-constructed common ground.

Vicki delayed coming to the health care facility for help with her pregnancy until near her sixth month. As a relatively young, unwed mother in a difficult family situation (an ex-husband—the father of her baby—with whom she is considering a reconciliation, a tiny child at home, a new, unplanned child on the way), this woman entered the health care encounter amidst considerable pressures and preconceptions. As a Native-American woman, cultural issues may have flavored her willingness to seek health care in the first place as well as her access to good health care information before her visit with these health caregivers (see Glenn, 1990). As with many women patients, Vicki could have benefited from discussions about her health and the wellness of herself and her unborn child. At the very least, Vicki could have been encouraged to participate more in her health care by receiving simple, short explanations about why information was important and what she could do now and in the future to facilitate her own well-being.

At this point, we would like to stress that the physician's assistant did recognize Vicki's face needs and multiplicity of identities later in the encounter by talking with her about Vicki's marital situation. Yet, as we observe early in this chapter and in our discussion of interactional framing in the previous one, relational activities must not be restricted to nonmedical asides. Interactants should not accept the notion that any part of the encounter is "medical" and somehow *not* about emergent relational and individual identities. The ability of caregivers and patients to collaboratively co-produce explanations is relationally, educationally, and medically consequential. Such explanations reflexively shape and constrain the ever-evolving relational dynamic, and the interactional co-orientation (or lack thereof) to caregiver and patient outlooks, identities, and commonalities impact the potentiality of patient education during health care encounters.

Like Excerpt 18, Excerpt 22 exemplifies how explanations can be co-accomplished as interactive patient education, wherein the patient's viewpoints become integral catalysts for how this caregiver describes medical issues. In the following exchange, the same physician's assistant at the Native-American health care facility interacts with "Tina," a woman who has come for an annual gynecologic examination and refill on birth control pills and who reveals that she has recurrent vaginal discharge.

Excerpt 22:

```
 1   C:   and you say you're having (.) is this unusual discharge
 2        (.) or is it just normal for you?
 3   P:   well (.) I'm beginning to wonder cause I I've always had
 4        discharge (.) but it's always been problems of yeast
 5        infection also
 6   C:   okay (.) does this seem yeasty to you? You know you've=
 7   P:   =umhum=
 8   C:   had it before so you know
 9   P:   yeah
10   C:   does it seem
11   P:   sort of (.) well (.) at one time it did and then it just
12        sorta went on its merry way (laughs)
13   C:   okay
```

14 P: and never did completely clear up
15 C: okay (.) the yeast never cleared up?
16 P: no ((indistinguishable)) Raylyn was treating it and it
17   went away and the it just (.) all of a sudden problems
18   getting rid of it
19 C: okay (.) how old are you?
20 P: twenty four
21 C: How many babies have you had?
22 P: one
23 C: okay (.) have you had any miscarriages or abortions?
24 P: one
25 C: okay (.) miscarriage or abortion?
26 P: abortion
27 C: okay (.) now (.) are you itchy? (.) >instances of<
28   [itching]
29 P: [every] every (.) now an then<=
30 C: =every >now an then< (.) so it >kind ov< (.) co:mes hhh
31   (.) an goes away=
32 P: =yah (.1)
33 C: okay (.2) now (.1) Tina (.) we a:lways >have uh<
34   discha:rge (.1) hhh I think women get mis (.) hhh
35   misunderstand (.) >when you have< (.) hhh discharge i:z
36   no:rmal (.) >to have< discharge (.)
37 P: mmhmm (.)
38 C: hhh (.) the sa:me >kind ov< tissue (.) hhh >well um< tha
39   same< (.) >kind ov< skin (.) >thatz inside< our vagina
40   (.) >iz tha< (.) sa:me >kind ov< skin thatz >inside
41   your< mouth (.)
42 P: wohawha=
43 C: =if you >take your< tongue (.2) >and you< feel it=
44 P: =mmhmm (.)
45 C: okay? (.1) and you >put your< finger (.) inside your<
46   vagi:na (.) hhh >itz tha< (.) >itz tha< same thing (.)
47   hhh you've got >little tiny< ce:llz (.) they're called
48   (.) go:blet cellz (.) they're they're uh special (.)
49   glandz that >secrete tha< saliva ta >keep your< mouth
50   dry (.) hhh (.) >if we< walked around (.) an our mouth
51   waz (.) waz u:m wazn't we:t (.) waz dry all da:y (.) an
52   we >want it ta be< wet (.) tha same thing with our
53   vagina (.) itz normal >to have uh< wetness (.1) hhh >in
54   your< vagina (.) otherwise (.) >it would< hurt to walk=
55 P: =hh kay=
56 C: =hh kay? (.) or (.) >really hurt ta< have sex (.) hhh

```
57        bu:t (.) uh discharge >thatznot< no:rmal (.) iz one
58        thatz (.1) got uh lot ov(.) it (.1) >uh itch< (.) >uh
59        bad< sme:ll (.) an odor (.2) >or any < (.) huh sticky
60        color (.) okay? hhh (.) >so we'll< check (.) >it
61        sounds< like you do: have one (.) but >itz normal< (.)
62        ta ha:ve >some dis<charge (.)
63   P:   okay
64   C:   >I think< (.) >alot ov< women think (.) oh (.) >my God< I
65        discharged (.) I >must have< an infection=
66   P:   =yah=
67   C:   =but (.) itz not (.1) >are you< using any >kind ov< birth
68        control (.) >right now<?
```

The physician's assistant begins by demonstrating an appreciation and respect for Tina's familiarity with her body and bodily functions. She asks for Tina's opinion about whether or not the discharge is "unusual" or "normal" in lines 1 and 2, marking her assumption that Tina could distinguish what was "unusual" or "normal" for her. Upon learning that Tina has a history of yeast infections, the physician's assistant probes to determine if Tina thinks that her present discharge resembles her past yeast infections. Tina responds indirectly, noting that her prior problems with yeast infection were never really resolved, but she never really answers whether or not the present discharge seems like those previous experiences with yeast infections.

However, instead of pursuing a more specific response from Tina or of offering clarification or information about yeast infections at that point, the physician's assistant says, "okay (.) how old are you?" in line 19. She proceeds to move away from the talk about the yeast infection to gain information about Tina's history with pregnancies in lines 19 through 26. Notably, the "okay" that begins her abrupt shift in line 19 works in a similar manner to the ones that were discussed near the end of Chapter 3—a swift change of topic initiated by the caregiver without reason or attention to the immediately prior subject of conversation. The physician's assistant offers no rationale for why the issue of pregnancies should be interactionally relevant or important now and gives no closure to their talk about potential yeast infections. With "okay" in line 27, the physician's assistant leaps from talk about Tina's pregnancy history back to talk about the discharge, yet again, without any reasoning or any exegesis about the relevance of the two seemingly unrelated topics.

These transitions from one topic to another without any accounting or connecting by the physician's assistant or without any questioning or commenting by the patient intensifies asymmetry in terms of control of the interaction and in terms of the knowledge differential. The very nature of such transitions reflexively deters co-orientation to the encounter as a team-like, partnership relational dynamic. To co-accomplish a partnership, interactants must collaborate, yet simultaneously and paradoxically, collaboration inherently conflicts with continual yet mundane instances of interactional asymmetry (i.e., "okay"-like transitions).

Unlike the other exchanges that already have been detailed in this section, however, the physician's assistant mandates such a shift to the prior discussion of the discharge to provide information. Also unlike those other exchanges, the physician's assistant revisits the discharge issue in a way that does not question the patient's perspective nor work reflexively to challenge the patient's potential competence as a viable partner in her own health care. Despite the perpetuation of asymmetry during the awkward transitions (which implicitly undermines the patient as a co-participant in the construction of the encounter), the ensuing explanation prompts and encourages Tina's active involvement in identifying potential health concerns.

In this interaction with Tina, the physician's assistant re-directs attention back to the discharge issue by asking a question about one of the symptoms of yeast infections—itching (lines 27–28). Tina suggests that she experiences itching "every now and then," and the physician's assistant repeats those words and then rephrases them "so it >kind ov< (.) co:mes an goes away." After Tina acknowledges that the physician's assistant has accurately depicted her discharge with "yah" in line 32, the physician's assistant indicates another transition by saying "okay," pausing, uttering "now," and again hesitating. She then commences with a lengthy talk about what constitutes "unusual" and "normal" discharge.

Although the physician's assistant starts the entire discussion with a question that presumes mutual knowledge and understanding of types of discharge, the ensuing discussion reveals that Tina really lacks a complete grasp of how to tell whether or not her discharge is potentially troublesome or not. Thus, the physician's assistant confronts the awkward task of giving Tina information while not threatening aspects of Tina's face because she has already implicitly suggested that Tina should be well-versed in making these distinctions, as someone who has a history of yeast infections. Notably, the physician's assistant could have avoided the next part of the interaction by noting "well, we'll check you out now" or "it doesn't sound like a yeast infection to me," thus progressing with the examination without explaining the differences nor empowering Tina to identify what is occurring in her body.

Yet, she opts to take a few minutes to educate Tina, to help her to understand. She begins by immediately referring to her and Tina with the inclusive pronoun, "we," fellow women who experience similar types of processes with their bodies, a practice that she continues throughout this description of what constitutes "normal discharge" (see lines 50 and 62). As we observe in Chapter 3, references to commonalities facilitate a bridging of the diverse array of identities, goals, and backgrounds between two individuals. In this case, the "we" and the link between "fellow women" work to diffuse, albeit not eliminate, possible embarrassment about talking and knowing about a very personal bodily function. Because Tina's complex set of intermingled identities includes participation as a "real" or "viable" member of the Native-American culture as well as preconceptions about what constitutes being a "lady" or a "respectable woman" in the Anglo-dominated, mainstream U.S. culture, she likely has some degree of reticence about discussing such issues. Thus, although such a discussion is medically important and relevant, this type of interaction can be more than just a little awkward—it can violate or disconfirm aspects that are integral to Tina's conception of who she is and who she wants to be, given her diverse, perhaps even conflicting, cultural and societal ties. However, by initiating this talk as a "fellow woman"—not someone from a different culture, not an authority figure who can pass judgment, not a stranger who she has just met—the physician's assistant facilitates a "just-between-you-and-me" type of interaction with a focus on something that they both experience.

The physician's assistant then promptly addresses the possible face threat stemming from providing a description of something that she has previously inferred that Tina already knows and potentially should know. She normalizes the misunderstanding by noting that she thinks women misunderstand that some discharge is normal, *not* that Tina misunderstood, not that Tina was ignorant (lines 34–36). The physician's assistant does not proceed accusingly ("why didn't you just tell me that you didn't know?") or condescendingly ("since you don't know, let me tell you"). Instead, her approach artfully allows her to excuse Tina's own lack of understanding on this issue; Tina becomes like most—or at least other—women who potentially misinterpret the meaning of discharge.

However, the physician's assistant never comes out and directly says that Tina has misunderstood or misinterpreted anything. Hence, when Tina responds with "mmhmm" to the physician's assistant's opening comments, she does not do so inappropriately; the physician's assistant cracks a door for her to continue to "play along" as a knowing other in this talk about women in general, not Tina in particular (even though, of course, there would be no reason for the interaction if Tina was indeed such a "knowing other.")

The physician's assistant continues with the description by noting that the mouth and the vagina have the same sort of skin. Although references simply to the skin in the vagina might have been embarrassing, the physician's assistant makes the comparison between that skin—in a private, concealed part of the body—to the mouth—a much more socially acceptable topic of discussion. She moves between the two, observing similarities and integrating a reference to one very acceptable practice—touching the tongue—versus one that might well be taboo—touching the vagina. However, she does so to advance the argument that the two body parts use similar fluids and that those fluids are vital and necessary in even walking around in everyday life. By discussing them as normal and essential, the physician's assistant supports her initial claim that discharge can be normal while also engaging in multifaceted facework and facilitating identification between fellow women.

In line 57, the physician's assistant starts to make the delineation between "normal" and "not normal" discharge. She tells Tina that discharge which is not normal involves itching, an unpleasant smell, a "sticky" color, thus providing her with information about how to identify for herself what she is experiencing. Yet, she offers this explanation by, again, revisiting the face needs of the patient. The physician's assistant observes that she will examine Tina for a yeast infection, commenting that ">it sounds< like you do: have one" (lines 60–61) but again reiterating that some discharge is normal. She even suggests, once more, that "a lot of" women react to discharge by assuming that they have some form of infection (lines 64–65). Hence, the physician's assistant makes Tina's reaction a common one, a legitimate one— something that others think, not just that "ignorant" or "stupid" people conclude. In so doing, the physician's assistant lays the groundwork for limiting face threats in the event that Tina does not have a yeast infection.

Through the relational activities of facework and identification, the explanation ensues in a manner that attends to the patient's multiplicity of identities, thus making that information accessible to her, to her lived reality. (In addition, reflexively, the nature of that explanation also contributes to the co-achievement of facework and identification.) As opposed to the other examples that have been provided in this section, this explanation simultaneously and reflexively attends to the patient's need to know and to the patient's array of identities and face concerns.

Through the giving of information in this manner, the caregiver treats the patient as a partner, as someone who can participate in her own care, not as someone to be dismissed. Yet interestingly, the patient tends to contribute little to the co-accomplishment of the explanation. Paradoxically, although the information empowers her to be a participant, the structure of the dissemination of information works to perpetuate the same asymmetry that permits caregiver-dictated abrupt topic shifts. Monologue-like explanations—even those that seemingly refer to patient perspectives—still leave the patient voice silent, with all-too-brief dialogue between the interactants and insufficient indications of how patients interpret and plan to integrate knowledge into their lived realities. The giving of information does not necessarily equate learning.

INITIATING AND REINFORCING PARTICIPATION

In 1984, Fisher compared doctor–patient discourse with teacher–student interactions, contending that doctors, like teachers, tend to control what transpires during exchanges. She suggested that doctors, like teachers, are "active and dominant" whereas patients, like students, are "passive and dependent" (Fisher, 1984, p. 201). In the previous portion of this chapter, we argue that caregivers need to offer explanations; however, we now want to go further by maintaining that the process of patient education can and must involve more of a conversation than a lecture. Building on the work of scholars in education, we suggest that education in the health care context ought not consist of a one-way model of information requests and then information dissemination. Instead, in this section, we elaborate on our earlier description of a preliminary "paradigm of interactive learning" in the health care context (see Ragan, Beck, & White, 1995) which suggests that active learning empowers patients.

Kolb (1984) offered a model of learning that embraces the lived realities and active involvement of students. Kolb maintained that uni-directional models do not adequately depict the complexity of the learning process; instead, he observed that people grasp new ideas by experimenting with them, wrestling with them, not simply soaking those ideas in like a passive sponge. As such, Kolb (1984, p. 21) viewed learning as processual and experiential, noting that "knowledge" is emergent and co-created, not pre-defined and absolute. Kolb's learning model serves as an impetus for creative re-inventions of teaching wherein teachers serve as facilitators and students actively engage in the co-construction of the educational process (see, e.g., Kendall, 1990; Kraft & Swadener, 1994).

We believe that Kolb's (1984) conception of learning can be enlightening and valuable as a point of departure for a re-thinking of the patient education process during caregiver–patient interactions, especially in light of the complexities of the postmodern era. As discussed in more detail in Chapter 2, caregivers and patients come together for brief snippets of time in their respective lives, bringing with them a plethora of potentially conflicting identities and fragmented connections to diverse collections of others. They enter the room with an eclectic assortment of material from a variety of sources, and they confront the frustration of the inherent irreconcilability of their ideas, perspectives, and orientations.

Without "a" truth to be attained "out there, somewhere," caregivers cannot stand on a medical pulpit and preach "a" gospel for well-being, nor can patients afford to quelch their dissonance and implicitly say "amen" to messages that do not quite seem to fit their situations, their unique yet fragmented identities, their preferences for relational dynamics. The scatteredness of the postmodern era defies such simplicity. One course of action cannot be served in a "cookie-cutter" manner to patients. Patients assume a vast range of different shapes, and, to enhance the conundrum for patients and caregivers, the complexity of each patient's composite of identities does not permit static, singular representation or treatment.

Thus, as caregivers and patients strive to share and learn, it cannot constitute an uncomplicated dispensing–consuming exchange. The chaos and

turmoil of the era, combined with the knowledge differential between caregivers and patients, renders the assumption of co-understanding and shared
perspectives and interpretations naive. Only through an interactive, collaborative process can caregivers and patients engage in an active, reciprocal
process of sharing, assimilating, and demonstrating interpretations and co-
orientations to information.

However, as we have observed thus far, patients who do voice their
opinions, concerns, and ideas venture into potentially risky interactional
territory. Although the health caregivers who participated in our research
projects interacted much more openly, affirmingly, and symmetrically with
their patients than we would expect based on our review of previous research
on health care interactions (see Chapter 1), we still found examples of
disconfirmation of patient participation (see Excerpt 16 in particular). In this
part of the chapter, we explore how health caregivers and patients can
interactionally co-facilitate patient participation in discussions about health
care, resulting in an interactive orientation to patient education.

In Excerpt 23, the physician's assistant at the Native-American health care
facility begins a pelvic examination on a patient. This patient ("Clara"), who
is seeking a refill on birth control pills, refers to her health care practices
throughout her encounter with the physician's assistant although the physician's assistant does little to prompt her to make such disclosures. Although
the physician's assistant does respond to Clara, she remarks only minimally,
a finding that is consistent with Jones' (1994, in press) work on assessments.

Excerpt 23:

1	C:	Okay (.) why don't you go ahead and scoot down toward me
2		(.) by the way (.) I didn't feel any abnormal lumps on
3		your breasts
4	P:	I always try to check mine
5	C:	good (.) good
6	P:	at the house (.) always (.) and I'll try to check them
7		myself
8	C:	good
9	P:	and if I feel anything (.) usually (.) I'm laying crooked
10		or something
11	C:	right (.) if you feel anything abnormal or see anything
12		abnormal (.) you want to get it checked too
13	P:	umhum
14	C:	you're still real young to get cancer of the breast but
15		it's a good health habit to get into
16	P:	see (.) I don't smoke (.) so I don't like cigarettes
17	C:	yeah (.) good
18	P:	so I'm real (.) I'll (.) I'll (.) about once every two

```
19          weeks or so I lay there in bed (.) flat like they
20          showed me how the first time
21    C:    right
22    P:    and I check my breasts (.)
23    C:    okay (.) that's good (.) feel a little pressure here on
24          the back wall (.) have you ever had problems with
25          urinary infection (.) infections of the bladder?
26    P:    no
```

In lines 1 through 3, the physician's assistant prepares to begin the pelvic examination and mentions, seemingly as an afterthought, that she "didn't feel any abnormal lumps" during her inspection of Clara's breasts. The prefacing of the remark with "by the way" and positioning of it as Clara moved toward the physician's assistant for another type of physical examination marks the breast issue as less than important. The physician's assistant does not describe what constitutes an "abnormal lump"; she does not inquire about the patient's understanding or knowledge of breast lumps and breast examinations; she does not reinforce the importance of self-examinations (which should be done in addition to annual visits with health caregivers).

When the physician's assistant presents her findings to Clara, she only cracks the door for interaction with Clara about this issue; she does not invite it. Yet, Clara tries to push herself through that sliver of an opening with a self-disclosure that demonstrates her awareness of self-examinations (line 4). The physician's assistant affirms Clara's disclosure, but she does so briefly with "good (.) good" (line 5). Clara continues in lines 6 through 7, reiterating that "I'll try to check them myself." Again, the physician's assistant responds with a simple "good."

The physician's assistant opts not to explore what Clara looks for as she "checks" them herself. She does not attempt to determine and clarify any misunderstandings, any misconceptions. The physician's assistant's lack of clarification implies that she assumes that Clara can tell the difference between what is and is not ordinary, without any evidence to support such a belief.

Although the physician's assistant does not ask, Clara volunteers more details about her examinations, noting that "usually," if she has felt something suspicious, she has just been "laying crooked or something" (lines 9–10). The physician's assistant affirms that statement with "right," yet she adds, again briefly, that Clara should "get it checked too" (lines 11–12).

Throughout this interaction, the physician's assistant's assessments of Clara's disclosures are limited, offering few specifics about why Clara's behavior is "good" or reinforcing what Clara should do and feel during examinations. Such assessments fit with Jones' (1994, in press) conclusion that caregivers do not routinely verbally react to patient disclosures of positive health behaviors. The exception in this exchange occurs in lines 14 through

15 when the physician's assistant compliments Clara on this "good health habit to get into" even though Clara is "still real young to get cancer of the breast."

However, when Clara goes on to note another health practice that should legitimately be treated as positive ("I don't smoke"), the physician's assistant once more only says "yeah (.) good," contributing little in the way of reaction or reinforcement. Even after Clara returns to the description of her self-breast examinations in lines 18 through 20 and 22, the physician's assistant merely utters "right" (line 21) and "okay (.) that's good" (line 23), before moving on to the next topic.

In short, although Clara attempts to present herself as a partner, as a knowledgeable patient, as a person who is concerned about her wellness, the physician's assistant does little to facilitate those self-presentations, to acknowledge the multiplicity of Clara's identities, and to perpetuate Clara's partnership-like initiatives. The facts that she does self-examinations and tries to engage in positive health practices are important to Clara, yet the physician's assistant implicity dismisses them, treating them as minutely significant. The physician's assistant does not fully seize the moment wherein she could help Clara through clarifications, reinforcements, and affirmation.

Conversely, Excerpt 24 provides a good example of an interaction in which the physician's assistant offers positive assessments and support for her patient's expressions of interest in, and desires to learn more about, her own situation. In this excerpt, she visits with "Alice," a pregnant woman, who has concerns about the positioning of her unborn child.

Excerpt 24:

```
 1   P:   Well (.) I was wondering (.) too (.) if it's lying sidewards
 2          (.) is my uterus ((unintelligible)) to go all the way up
 3          (.) like this?
 4   C:   unhun
 5   P:   I have been reading about it (.)
 6   C:   have you? good (.) did you get some good material to read?
 7          (.) I've got a good (.) an extra book there if you need
 8          one (.)
 9   P:   yeah (.) I'd like to read it (.)
10   C:   okay
11   P:   I'll bring it back next time I come (.)
12   C:   okay (.) no you can keep it (.)
13   P:   okay
```

Alice starts this exchange by noting that she's been "wondering" about whether the baby is "lying sidewards" and then asks directly whether it will "go all the way up (.) like this" (lines 1–3). The physician's assistant responds with "unhun" in line 4, again, a very limited response that contains sparse information or encouragement for Alice to think about this situation.

In line 5, however, Alice contends that she has not just "wondered" about it; she has "been reading about it." The physician's assistant shows some surprise with "have you?" and says "good" in line 6. However, unlike Excerpt 23, the physician's assistant attends to Alice's overt indication of interest further by asking her if she obtained "some good material to read" (line 6) and then by offering her "a good (.) an extra book there if you need one" (lines 7–8). In so doing, the physician's assistant demonstrates her interest in and support of Alice's pursuit of understanding. Furthermore, she provides Alice with a source of more information.

Notably, the physician's assistant does so while recognizing potential face concerns. The question about Alice's initial choice of reading material could threaten Alice's identity as one who can competently select a book with quality content. The physician's assistant rephrases her offer from a "good" book (perhaps as opposed to Alice's choice) to "an extra book," one that could be referred to in addition to, an enrichment of, Alice's book. The physician's assistant avoids sounding condescending and critical. Instead, she extends the book to Alice; if Alice decides that she needs one, she can access it. In this case, the offering and subsequent accepting of the extra reading material enables the interactants to co-produce a collaborative effort, an interactive one. They engage in a dialogue wherein the physician's assistant serves as a facilitator, not simply a person who gives "answers," and the patient participates as a partner, not simply a person who passively receives those "answers."

Furthermore, this exemplar of interactive learning illustrates a both–and solution to the conundrum of patient learning in a tight time context. The interactional means through which the physician's assistant and Alice address her educational goals do not unnecessarily elongate the encounter; in fact, the physician's assistant equips Alice to learn more about her pregnancy without spending time during the health care encounter. Yet, in so doing, she validates and promotes Alice's desire to do so. The physician's assistant empowers Alice to take on responsibility for gaining and assimilating that information while making it clear that she can be a helpful resource person.

Notably, this approach fits well with the postmodern condition. Because there are no absolute, pre-defined answers to be given, Alice positions herself as someone who wants to learn for herself, to sort through material within the context of her complicated lived reality. The physician's assistant can then assist Alice in understanding and interpreting that information in an interactive, dyadic manner—not a lecture-like monologue. Through this co-orientation to patient education, they reflexively permit the realization of aspects of identity beyond one who knows and one who does not, making

the knowledge differential less distinct, the potentiality of the multiplicity
of selves more attainable.

As in Excerpt 24, Excerpt 25 illustrates interactive learning as the physician's assistant and "Margaret," another pregnant patient, jointly co-produce
co-definitions as they converse about dietary issues. The physician's assistant
acknowledges Margaret's understanding as Margaret also reifies the physician's assistant's assertions of what should count as important and salient
to her pregnancy.

Excerpt 25:

```
 1   C:   I want you to re:st (.) re:st (.) as much as you can do (.)
 2        is just re:st (.) hhh when >you go< home (.) >you tell<
 3        your husband you make dinner honey (.) hhh you take care
 4        of me (.) . . . I need >to set< down (.) I need >to rest<
 5        (.)
 6   P:   mmkay (.)
 7   C:   and >get down< (.) watch your sodium (.) the salt=
 8   P:   =right=
 9   C:   =potato chips (.) hhh hidden salt (.) ketchup (.) mustard
10        (.) pickles (.) >pickle relish< (.) all that stuff is
11        lo:aded with sodium (.)
12   P:   che:ese (.)
13   C:   che:ese (.)
14   P:   calcium (.) >I know<
15   C:   right (.) calcium (.) but milk? (.)
16   P:   I know (.) [I've been drink]in milk=
17   C:              [that's the better] =that's the better
18        alternative (.) yah (.) we just want uh (.) healthy
19        healthy baby (.) >and we want< you healthy too (.) hhh
20        your hematocrit? are you taking your iron tablets now?
21   P:   hhh ye:s (.) ha ha (.)
22   C:   okay (.) your hematocrit >is up< a little bit (.) at
23        >thirty five< percent (.)
24   P:   which (.) I don't under?=
25   C:   =okay (.) well (.) the numbers (.) okay (.) >let's see< the
26        last time we >did a< hematocrit on you (.) it was
27        >forty percent< (.) and that was in January (.)
28   P:   o:h (.) >for the< diabetes?=
29   C:   =no no (.) that's >for the< for the red blood cell count
30        (.)
31   P:   oh (.)
32   C:   okay (.) >so it's gone down< (.) okay (.) anemia (.) okay=
33   P:   =mmhmm=
```

```
34   C:   =women develop anemia (.) hhh >often times< (.) when they
35        get pregnant (.) because (.) hh they don't have enough
36        ir:on (.) for their red blood cells (.) because your
37        body's (.) making red blood cells hhh (.) >for the< baby=
38   P:   =right=
39   C:   =>the baby's< (.) making its blood cells really (.) but (.)
40        the baby takes iron from you (.)
41   P:   right
```

The physician's assistant begins this excerpt by directing Margaret to get rest (lines 1–5), and Margart agrees with "mmkay" in line 6. The physician's assistant continues with another directive "watch your sodium," doing a self-corrective to "salt," a word that may be more accessible to the patient in line 7. However, instead of "mmkay," Margaret agrees by saying "right" in line 8, indicating her familiarity with this need.

As such, Margaret starts to assert herself as someone who has either had this discussion with a caregiver before or who has had some kind of experience with this type of dietary issue before. In essence, she presents herself as a knowing participant, as a co-teller—co-constructor—of the description that ensues. The potential interactional problem here is that interactants normally do not repeat information to others who share that prior knowledge without making reference to that sharedness and offering an account for the re-telling (see Mandelbaum, 1987). The physician's assistant does not commence this exchange with any reference to Margaret's familiarity with what she intends to say (i.e., "I know that we've been through this before, but . . ." or "I know that you must have heard all about this in your prior pregnancies, but . . .").

Although Margaret says "right" in line 8, the physician's assistant does not treat that as a sign that Margaret may be positioning herself as a person who already knows what foods contain salt. The physician's assistant proceeds to list a few items that are high in sodium (lines 9–11). In line 12, though, Margaret adds "cheese" to the list, and the physician's assistant affirms that response by repeating and further emphasizing "che:ese" in line 13. Margaret then extends her demonstration of dietary knowledge by raising the issue of "calcium" and asserting "I know" in line 14.

In line 15, the physician's assistant acknowledges that calcium is an important issue but introduces a possible clarification in the form of a question or alternative: Milk can provide calcium without the salt that is in cheese, another source of calcium. By raising milk as a question, the physician's assistant now alludes to the possibility that Margaret understands about the need for calcium and the usefulness of milk, unlike her previous utterances where she interactionally displays the assumption that Margaret does not have that information. Margaret perpetuates the co-treatment of herself as a knowing other by responding with "I know" and "I've been drinkin milk" in line 16. She then offers the positive assessment that "that's the better (.) that's the better alternative" and reiterates that these issues are important for both the baby and for Margaret (lines 17–19).

Although the physician's assistant could have started this sequence by asking Margaret about her awareness of dietary information, she opts not to do so. Thus, she begins without a basis for cultivating a common ground, a shared understanding, and her inaccurate guess sets up a situation wherein aspects of Margaret's identity become at risk. The physician's assistant does adjust, facilitating and recognizing Margaret's orientation to the information as someone who also knows. If she had just forged ahead with her talk about the dietary concerns without responding to Margaret's level of understanding, the physician's assistant might have uttered words that contained information, but patient education (and likely, medical outcomes) may have been hindered by the lack of attention to relational goals. Margaret could well have felt disconfirmed by the implicit dismissal of that part of her identity and her preference to be treated in a particular way. Because relational, medical, and educational goals all intertwine, the implications could have been significant for Margaret's perspective on how well this caregiver can respond to her specific needs, to her lived reality and for Margaret's subsequent willingness to trust the recommendations of someone who obviously does not work to identify with her.

In line 20, the physician's assistant refers to another issue, "hematocrit," and asks whether Margaret takes her iron pills. Margaret says "yes" with a brief chuckle, and the physician's assistant moves on to tell her about the results of a blood test. She does so by referring to the technical name instead of the lay name, iron, and talking about percentages without offering information. Notably, because Margaret has positioned herself as a knowing participant and the physician's assistant has oriented to Margaret as such, explanations could be viewed as unnecessary and perhaps even condescending by the physician's assistant. However, unlike before, Margaret now indicates that she does not understand this particular subject.

The physician's assistant initially tries to address Margaret's lack of understanding by giving her a perspective on the numbers, referring to the results of a previous test (lines 25–27). Yet, when Margaret voices her candidate interpretation of the reason for the tests (i.e., "diabetes") in line 28, the physician's assistant steps back even further to explain what the test measured (i.e., "the red blood cell count") in line 29. The physician's assistant then no longer assumes sharedness in terms of a co-orientation to this topic. She tells Margaret the implications of a lower test score ("anemia") in line 32 and then describes what causes this condition (lines 34–37). Interestingly, in lines 38 and 41, the patient responds with "right," again implying that she has some sort of familiarity. By this point, she may be referring to the recollection of prior knowledge. In any case, Margaret's earlier admission of confusion permits the physician's assistant to offer information without potential face threats due to repeated topics.

Through their collaborative engagement in this dialogue, Margaret and the physician's assistant permit the emergence of a co-constructed, shared understanding. They do so by reflexively attending to implicit and concurrent face concerns and by working with each other in terms of their complicated, multifaceted, preferred individual and relational identities. As Excerpts 24 and 25 suggest, interactive learning becomes possible through and contributes to a relational dynamic wherein the interactants co-achieve a partnership as part of their relational co-definition.

A REVIEW

We begin this chapter by reiterating our conviction that relational, educational, and medical goals intertwine and that the interactional activities that contribute to one aspect of goal work inherently impacts and works reflexively to facilitate or deter the other simultaneous goals that caregivers and patients bring to and advance during health care encounters. Hence, as the exemplars in this chapter illustrate, the way in which explanations occur necessarily contributes to the concurrent and continual re-shaping of the emergent relational dynamic, and that relational dynamic frames how information gets co-constructed by interactants.

For example, when caregivers and patients treat each other as partners for some fragment of time when they are together (as in Excerpt 25), the co-accomplishment of knowledge and understanding occurs much differently than the monologue-like telling of information from earlier excerpts in the chapter. The critical difference involves more of an active co-construction than a passive giving then receiving of "facts."

As we stress, given the postmodern era and the knowledge differential between health care participants, caregivers and patients can no longer assume that they share interpretations of such "facts" nor that "facts" constitute static entities to be grasped. We echo Gadamer's position that interpretation must be construed as temporal and emergent. In so doing, we suggest that dialogues about medical data should consist of re-interpretations, not the assumption that only one way exists to ascertain meaning. By viewing patient learning as interactive, caregivers and patients may co-orient to knowledge as fluid, not preordained, and they may collaboratively produce interpretations in light of their lived realities, their multiplicity of diverse windows on the world.

This stance on interactive patient learning poses potential implications for medical goals as well as relational ones. By co-defining patients as partners and active participants, caregivers and patients reflexively empower patients and give them at least partial responsibility for medical choices and outcomes. Furthermore, the integration of patient perspectives during a dialogue affords caregivers a heightened appreciation for patient orientation to the encounter, health practices, and shared information. As we discuss in the next chapter, the co-achievement of a collaborative partnership— wherein caregivers and patients co-orient to a multiplicity of identities, goals and perspectives as well as co-construct some common ground of under- standing—underlies the potentiality for accomplishing medical goals.

The Co-Accomplishment of Medical Goals

Around 4 p.m. on a rainy afternoon, I was shadowing doctors and nurses in the emergency room at one of the hospitals where I was collecting ethnographic data. Perhaps because of the rain, the emergency room was overflowing with people from car crashes and other accidents. When the emergency medical crew brought in "Mallory," I followed one of the female nurses into the tiny examining room and listened to one of the male emergency crew members quickly tell the nurse about Mallory's case: 14 years old, stole some stuff from a mall jewelry store, told parents, parents forcing her to return stuff, swallowed some of mom's sleeping pills instead, informed mom and dad when she did, conscious when picked up about half an hour after consuming pills, vitals steady. The nurse nodded and, for the first time, glanced at Mallory.

The girl lay on the hospital bed where the emergency crew had moved her from the stretcher. She did not look at any of the people who were talking about her, treating them as invisible—just as they seemingly failed to recognize her. She stared at her hands, noticeably absent of any rings or adornment. The nurse walked over to Mallory and placed her hand on Mallory's wrist to get a pulse. She proceeded to obtain Mallory's vital signs while talking sporadically with the emergency crew. "Are the parents on their way?" she asked. "Yeah," the one crew member responded, "the mom was pretty freaked. It seems that this one's been kind of a problem. Just got out of court-mandated counseling after another incident. Not sure what to do with her." "Oh my . . . hhh okay, we'll keep an eye out for them," the nurse said.

As I sat on the chair in front of Mallory's bed, I experienced feelings of disbelief and dismay about their lack of regard for this teen's feelings. They interacted about her as though she was not in the room, as though her problems, fears, anxieties, and apprehensions meant nothing. I wanted to stand beside her, take her hand, assure her that she would be all right, and, ever-the-"mom" myself, tell her that no situation was bad enough for this. However, I quickly quelched that urge. First, I reminded myself that I wanted to observe how these health caregivers and patients interact during such stressful encounters, and second, I re-realized that Mallory obviously had another view of how "bad" a situation could be and what choices were "good" or "not so good," given the context of her complicated life.

As I watched the emergency medical crew member and the nurse continue their conversation and then leave the room, I still could not fathom how these health caregivers could ignore Mallory's presence in the room, not adjusting their remarks to include her in the interaction, talking about her not with her. I could not comprehend how they could maintain a tunnel-vision on medical tasks without verbally recognizing the underlying but overwhelmingly relevant nonmedical task issues (i.e., the circumstances surrounding Mallory's decision to swallow the tablets, the extent to which Mallory desired to live, the paradoxical struggle for Mallory as she juxtaposed her desire to know what would happen next with her own actions that thrust her into this tentative and precarious position).

As we have observed throughout this book, during even the most ideal of health care encounters, caregivers and patients struggle with the unresolvable tension of a multiplicity of potentially conflicting concerns, goals, and identities—individual and relational. The interplay of those issues can inhibit the ability of interactants to present themselves (and to position themselves in terms of others) in preferred manners, resulting in an interactional climate wherein threats to aspects of interactant identity can evolve. Mallory found herself in a particularly face-threatening situation.

Unlike patients in the gynecologic setting (wherein patients do not "want" the examination but yet they undergo one for the early detection of disease), Mallory catapulted herself into this potentially frightening and intimidating scenario. She opted to do something contradictory to staying "well," yet ironically, she was now here seeking care. Hence, to offer Mallory an "out" for any embarrassment or awkwardness that she felt about her situation, her caregivers would have had to either condone her choice to consume the pills or come up with some other very creative way of accounting for or excusing her behavior. They chose not to do so. Mallory continued to stare at her hands as the caregivers moved around her. No one mentioned the "elephant in the room" (the suicide attempt), yet that beast crowded and cramped everyone and everything in that tiny cubicle. It was invisible albeit glaringly obvious as all carefully tiptoed around it.

The male emergency room doctor came into Mallory's cubicle about 10 minutes later. He scanned her chart, examined her quickly, and said, "We need to get these pills out of your system before they do permanent damage." Mallory spoke for the first time. "Do I need to have my stomach pumped?" she asked. "Yes, we need to absorb the pills before they hurt you any further. As it is, we can't know the extent of the damage until later," the doctor said, turning to the nurse and giving more detailed instructions. Mallory started to cry. "Will it hurt?" she asked. "Well, it's not comfortable," the doctor said. "Can I be asleep?" she inquired. "No, you need to be awake," the doctor responded. "Can you give me something to make it not hurt?" she pleaded. The doctor paused, shaking his head, and said softly, "I think that you've taken enough for today."

As they prepared the room for the procedure, the nurse glanced at me and asked if I wanted to wait outside. I indicated that I did not want to be in the way, and she noted that I would not be any trouble; however, she called the procedure "disturbing" and wished to forewarn me. I said that I wanted to stay. Hearing our talk from the nearby bed, Mallory sobbed still louder.

Throughout Mallory's first 20 minutes in the hospital, two emergency medical crew members, three nurses, one doctor, and two laboratory technicians entered her area and performed some sort of medical task (i.e., the reporting of the status of the case, the taking of vitals, the drawing of blood, the recommendation of procedures, and the preparation for those procedures). Yet, no one but the doctor spoke to Mallory at length, except to give her short commands: "sit up now," "lay down now," "need your arm." They focused on her body, not on the complex, multifaceted person who uses it as a vessel; no one explored Mallory's perspectives on the events at the hospital. No one attempted to explain to her what was going to occur. Instead, Mallory remained motionless in the hospital bed, watching the caregivers, tears streaming from her eyes. No one even made an effort to give her a tissue to wipe her runny nose.

Finally, the nurses indicated that they were ready to perform the procedure, putting on their gloves and picking up the necessary equipment. In essence, they needed to force a tube down Mallory's nose to her stomach, insert a chalk-like substance, wait for the substance to absorb the pills, and then flush the substance from her system. As one of the nurses held the tube close to Mallory's nose, she explained what was about to occur and offered Mallory some short tips on how to help the task advance quickly and efficiently (i.e., try not to vomit, try to remain calm). Mallory panicked and cried, "I don't want to do this. I don't want you to do this." The nurse put her hand on Mallory's arm, looked directly into her eyes, and said, "We *are* going to do this. You can make this easy on yourself or hard on yourself, but this *has* to happen."

She paused for a moment, looking at the girl's puffy, red eyes, her tear-stained cheeks, her runny nose, her tense and rigid body. "Let's get through this. Here, put your hands on the sides of the bed and squeeze as hard as you want. Focus on not throwing up. If you lose any, we have to add more, and it takes all the longer. Come on now. It'll be all right." Mallory slowly placed her hands on the rails, but, as the nurse started to insert the tube in her nose, she screamed, "noooo" and grabbed at the tube.

The other nurse took Mallory's hand and placed it back on the rail, and, for the first time, she massaged Mallory's shoulder. As the nurse with the tube tried again, the second nurse continued to rub Mallory's shoulder, to dab Mallory's nose, to let her know what would happen next, to talk to her about topics like the weather, and to note "that's a good job," "you're doing fine now," "breath now," "relax."

From the cringes that crossed Mallory's face from time to time, I could tell that the procedure caused her great discomfort. However, she responded to the coaching, only vomiting a little once and not panicking again. Although I doubt that Mallory could have avoided the procedure by protesting or physically fighting the nurses, I do believe that it would have been much harder on her if she had continued to verbally and bodily circumvent the procedure. We have no way of knowing how Mallory would have responded if the nurse had not reached out to her, attending to parts of her identity and face needs, giving her information, enabling her to participate as a partner in the difficult and painful process. However, as I sat in that bedside chair observing the co-accomplishment of the procedure, I witnessed a life-saving medical task that became more possible as the patient contributed to—not just cooperated with—the co-achievement of the pumping of the stomach. She did so within an emergent interactional dynamic that expanded to embrace her as a person with feelings, thoughts, preferences, and needs, not simply as a person who took some pills.

When I talked to my co-ethnographer (who is also a registered nurse) about my experience in the emergency room, I commented on my frustration with the health caregivers. She slowly nodded and remarked, "It's hard, ya know. We are busy attempting to save lives, and most of us have little patience with people who try to end their own by choice." As I reflected on that day in the emergency room, I could appreciate that perspective. On that day alone, I watched stretcher after stretcher carry people with dire injuries to surgery, and I silently noted the pain of their families as they anxiously kept vigil in the waiting room. For those caregivers to include Mallory in their day, within the chaotic context of those other patients who were fighting for their own lives, a lack of tolerance can be at least partially understood.

However, as we detail throughout this chapter, recognition of relational and educational goals does not constitute some nicety, some extra. Instead, attention to relational and educational goals can reflexively facilitate the very doing of medical tasks and the co-accomplishment of an array of medical goals. Even in cases of attempted suicide like Mallory's, relational communication cannot simply be ignored or dismissed. As we emphasize in Chapter 2, the disregard of Mallory's tears and the disconfirmation of her fears and her multiplicity of identities inherently contributes to and shapes the emergent relational dynamic. Although those caregivers might not have been trying to establish any kind of relationship with this particular patient, they reflexively did so anyway, and the medical consequences included a difficult and tentative start to an important medical procedure.

In this chapter, we focus on the interactional resources that can enhance caregiver and patient ability to collaboratively work toward two important medical goals—co-achieving medical tasks during the examination and co-defining of preferred health practices. Through a joint co-orientation to medical goals, the interactants permit a team-like, partnership-like approach to attaining preferred medical outcomes in mutually acceptable and beneficial manners. Furthermore, we demonstrate how the co-achievement of simultaneous relational and educational goals facilitates the co-accomplishment of medical ones. All activities play a part in how these sets of goals are or are not realized; all inherently and reflexively weave together, advancing, perpetuating, and reifying those activities and goals.

Co-Achieving of Medical Tasks

Certainly, not all medical procedures are as potentially painful as the one that Mallory faced; not all medical examinations are as potentially face-threatening as gynecologic exams. However, notably, we envision the doing of medical tasks as encompassing a range of physical and emotional discomfort, not being with pain or embarrassment or without them. As caregivers and patients work toward wellness and optimum health outcomes, they cannot bracket off medical tasks anymore than they can separate relational activities. Medical tasks take place as part of, and contribute to, the ever-emergent relational dynamic that evolves between, and because of, the particular interactants at the specific point in time. As we observed in Excerpt 21, the physician's assistant might have been attempting to obtain information about Vicki's weight, but the nature of the interaction had significant face implications that may not be discarded simply because the threat occurred in the context of a medical task (i.e., obtaining part of a patient's history).

Caregivers and patients may diffuse, although never eliminate, the asymmetry of medical tasks by taking a partnership co-orientation to procedures and examinations. In so doing, the task becomes less of something that is being "done to" a patient and more of something that the patient becomes intricately involved in co-accomplishing, thus advancing a number of concurrent goals. For example, in Mallory's case, the coaching by the second nurse enabled Mallory to focus on productive behaviors that were conducive to the examination instead of succumbing to her first impulse—to fight the procedure. As in coaching during natural childbirth, the encouragement and guides for involvement to patients from caregivers can ease and expediate examinations, difficult procedures, and so on. Such coaching also permits the reflexive co-emergence of aspects of a particular type of relational dynamic—a partnership between two individuals with fluid yet distinct identities who merge together to make a single event occur in a preferred manner.

Through artful interactional framing, caregivers and patients may meta-recognize the unpleasantness of some examinations and procedures. They can also collaboratively devise some way for patients to participate and/or to attend to the multifaceted nature of the activity. For example, in Excerpt 26, the nurse practitioner at the university health care facility verbally acknowledges the awkward nature of a pelvic examination and offers "Amanda" a quick tip on how to make the exam a bit easier.

Excerpt 26:

```
1    C:    now >I'm going ta relax<  your vaginal muscle with my
2          finger (.) okay? (.2) an this iz tha speculum (.3) a
3          little tender? (.) okay there ya go (.) okay (.) think
4          about relaxing that (.) >a little bit uncomfortable<
5          isn't it? (.)
6    P:    yah
7    C:    I'll try to be as >quick as I can<
```

The nurse practitioner informs Amanda about each increment of the procedure as she starts to do it, and notably, she involves Amanda by repeatedly seeking her involvement. She asks "okay?" in line 2 and "a little tender?" in line 3. Although Amanda does not verbally respond, the questions implicitly indicate the nurse practitioner's preference to recognize potential concerns and to include the patient in the co-construction of the activity. The nurse practitioner remarks on Amanda's participation by stating "there ya go" and then offering a gentle suggestion on how to make the examination easier for her in lines 3 and 4. However, as the nurse practitioner tells Amanda to "relax" a certain muscle, she also provides Amanda with an "out" if she cannot do so—the procedure is uncomfortable, thus making relaxing difficult. Following that reference to the admitted essence of the exam, the nurse practitioner further attends to Amanda's physical and emotional concerns by promising to be "as quick as I can."

As we discuss in Chapter 3, meta-recognitions of the patient's perspective can also occur through the collaborative co-achievement of shared laughter. In Excerpts 5 and 6, we detail how shared laughter provides caregivers and patients with an interactional means through which to address paradoxes of patient identities and to acknowledge multiple concurrent realities. In so doing, shared laughter enables caregivers and patients to co-achieve connectedness, contributing to and enhancing a multiplicity of simultaneous identities, activities, and goals.

This type of mutual attention to patient co-involvement in examinations and procedures reflexively facilitates a number of relational and medical goals. Caregivers and patients can achieve a common ground of shared understanding and perspective, thus contributing to trust, which simultaneously impacts the doing of the examination as well as the emergent relational dynamic. Such meta-recognitions constitute the type of interactional framing that we advance in Chapter 2—an integrated treatment of an event in light of the multiplicity of concurrent activities (not the accomplishing of one thing or another). Thus, the acknowledgment of patient discomfort is not some sort of unrelated aside; it reflexively becomes part of, as well as occurs through and during, particular medical activities *and* relational activities (i.e., identification and facework). The co-orientation permits the simultaneous realization of the patient as a person who is undergoing an examination, a person who is participating in the examination, and a person who has a multiplicity of identities and related face concerns. We stress here that such interactional framings allow all of this without unnecessarily elongating the encounter; if anything, they permit medical tasks to occur more efficiently and expediently. In the case of shared laughter, for example, Ragan (1990) observed that the integration of humor can serve a relaxation function, permitting the patient to reduce physical and emotional tension and to allow her body to be more conducive to examinations, especially gynecologic ones.

Co-Defining of Preferred Health Care Practices

As detailed in Chapter 1, an area of health communication that has garnered significant interest involves patient compliance with health care recommendations. As we come to this issue, however, we envision a much more murky model than practitioners recommending–patients complying. Our stance that recommendations must be collaboratively co-achieved extends far beyond the notion that patients will engage in positive health practices if they feel like they are part of decisions. We contend that the nature of patients' lives requires them to determine possible options with their caregivers (and vice versa) that will be workable, given the chaotic, scattered nature of their lived realities.

For example, I recently visited my ophthalmologist because my eye was infected. He examined me and prescribed a cream for my eyelid, which he directed me to use four times a day. While he was writing the prescription, I watched as my two children darted around the doctor's office—I had them with me because school was out and my sitter canceled. When the doctor told me that the cream would make my eye blurry for around a half an hour each time that I used it, I let out a half-hearted chuckle. With two very active children to watch, a book to finish, a house and four pets to care for, and a summer class to teach, there was no way that I could use the medication as directed. However, with all of those things on my mind and the tension of watching two bored children start to climb on expensive equipment in the office, I accepted the prescription, paid the bill, and left the office for the pharmacy. Fortunately, my eye was able to heal on the one dose a day that I was able to apply right before falling into bed.

Like myself and the active college student in Excerpt 12 in Chapter 3, most women lead lives that whip by at a frantic pace. The conundrum that most of us face stems from our sincere desire to solve our health care concerns that conflict with, yet are important because of, the tumultuous nature of our lives. Although not all situations permit caregivers to be as flexible and as accommodating as the one in Excerpt 12, attention to this dilemma—as well as to the multiplicity of goals and concerns *and* to the diversity and plethora of potentially conflicting information and perspectives—must occur for problems to be addressed and hopefully resolved. In the case of Nancy, the woman who voiced a desire for a Pap smear in Excerpt 4, the caregiver did not pursue the underlying reasons for Nancy's preference, nor did she explore possible misconceptions. As such, Nancy's medical goal was brushed aside.

However, the ongoing paradox is how caregivers can provide expert insight on a medical situation, which their patients pay good money to receive, while inviting and incorporating patient input. If caregivers are the experts, and patients spend their time, energy, and finances soliciting that expertise, how can both parties reconcile a greater involvement of patients and resolve multiple concurrent face issues (i.e., potential caregiver and patient awkwardness over making caregiver expertise problematic, conflicting aspects of patient identity—passive patient while active consumer, active consumer while busy person)?

We suggest that the answer lies in the reconceptualization of health care "answers," "recommendations," and "solutions" as emergent, temporal, and co-constructed, *not* pre-defined, static, and absolute. As we have noted throughout this volume, the overabundance of information has produced few certainties, and the postmodern condition precludes "a" reality amidst the fragmented, frazzled lives of people in the now ambiguous and tentative world. Hence, caregivers can offer their expertise as individuals who have a grasp of medical research and who come to encounters with medical training, but even that understanding cannot permit them to slice through the complexities of human bodies, souls, and lives to render simplistic, clear-cut solutions that fit each person. For that expertise to be realized as a resource, patients must contribute to the dialogue, providing caregivers with a hint of the context in which medical solutions must necessarily occur.

We have broached some interactional ways in which patients and caregivers may engage in dialogues as partners (see Chapters 3 and 4). However, we also recognize that, at some point, plans must be laid on the table for discussion, even in the most interactive of health care encounters. We suggest here that caregivers may continue to facilitate an interactive co-orientation to health care encounters by offering directives as suggestions. In each of the following examples, we demonstrate the intertangledness of the three types of goals that we identify in this book—relational, educational, and medical. We note how each reflexively contributes to, and gets enabled or deterred because of, the others.

In Excerpt 27, we return to Vicki, from Excerpts 15, 16, 17, and 21 in Chapter 4. Despite her earlier problems with the nurse and the physician's assistant, in this exchange Vicki and the physician's assistant discuss Vicki's marital situation. The physician's assistant provides input; however, she does so by couching this as something that Vicki might want to "think about."

Excerpt 27:

```
 1  C:   you might >think about< (.) out[side counseling]
 2  P:                                [well yah] (.)
 3  C:   >have you< done that? (.)
 4  P:   yah (.) we've been um (.1) working (.) >tryin ta< work
 5       things out for >tha past< three months (.) we've been
 6       (.) >tryin ta< get back together=
 7  C:   =uh uh (.4) cause >often times< (.1) those things >don't
 8       resolve< themselves >until they're< ta:lked abo:ut (.)
 9  P:   yah (.)
10  C:   >an you< can >talk about< your feelings (.) >and your<
11       rage (.) and >what you< expect from hi:m uh (.) hhh an
12       he >needs ta: (.) >ya know< (.) be >able ta< fulfill
13       your needs and you >need ta be< able ta hhh fulfill
14       hi:s hhh otherwise (.) just be >gettin back< together
15       hhh (.) >if you< don't resolve those pro:blems (.)
16       they'll all come back (.) >an they< (.) >need ta be<
17       talked about (.) an ya >need ta< (.) >be able ta< (.)
18       really (.) have those >out in tha< open hhh (.) now I
19       don't ask people >to reveal< a:ll feelings about
20       themselves (.) >but they< (.) >need ta< talk about
21       >some of< them
```

Although Vicki acknowledges that she might want to think about counseling, her response to the physician's assistant's more direct question ">have you< done that?" indicates that she has not yet sought such help. In line 7, the physician's assistant builds on her suggestion about counseling from line 1, picking up where she left off with that prior utterance. She then offers an explanation for that suggestion as well as raising a number of issues that Vicki should attempt to resolve with her husband before proceeding with a reconciliation.

Although Vicki responds minimally to the physician's assistant (perhaps in light of her prior exchanges with her), the physician's assistant's efforts in this case exemplify an intermingling of attention to patient education and to aspects of Vicki's identity as a wife and partner with her husband. Notably, Vicki's lack of participation undermines the physician's assistant's ability to ascertain whether or not her own lived reality as far as personal relationships rings true with Vicki's beliefs, preconceptions, and experiences. Yet, the offering of the recommendation as a suggestion rather than a command (i.e., "you *need* to do this") positions this as something that Vicki could choose to do, and by extension, implies that Vicki can decide for herself, as a competent person, whether she will act on the recommendation or not.

The argument might be made that caregivers have the luxury of phrasing directives as suggestions when they talk about something nonmedical. However, as we note in Excerpt 18 (Chapter 4) such an approach, combined with explanations, facilitates the reflexive co-accomplishment of relational, educational, and medical goals.

In Excerpts 28, 29, and 30, the physician's assistant at the Native-American health care facility responds to "Ellen's" concern about her cough. Ellen raised this issue with the nurse who took her history, and she refers to that conversation in Excerpt 28.

Excerpt 28:

```
1   P:   mmhmm (.4) she told me (.) u:m (.2) to te:ll yo:u also: (.)
2        >about tha< co:ld (.) >that I've< had (.) >I've had it
3        for< (.) almost (.) thre:e weeks (.) now
4   C:   okay (.)
5   P:   started >coughing up< uh >little blood< (.) last ni:ght
6   C:   okay (.6) birthdate?
```

In this excerpt, Ellen offers a presequence for the topic of the cough and, likely, her desires for the physician's assistant to examine the reason for her cough as well as to give her something for the cough. Ellen hesitantly initiates the issue after a lull in the conversation. She does so by citing a source, the nurse, who told her to tell the physician's assistant (line 1). Ellen's reliance on the nurse's credibility rather than her own indicates that Ellen perceives a status differential. (We would not likely hear Susan, the university professor from Chapter 3, depend on an outside source for legitimacy in advancing a concern.) When the physician's assistant does not respond right away,

Ellen notes that the cough has lingered for almost 3 weeks (line 3) and then that she even "started >coughing up< uh >little blood< (.) last ni:ght" (line 5). However, the physician's assistant does not pursue the presequence at that time, nor does she note that she will return to the subject. She merely says "okay" in line 6, pauses, and then asks for her birthdate.

Because we do not have access to videotaped data, we do not know whether or not the physician's assistant wrote the concern on the chart to return to it later. Although that is a possibility, even if it is the case, the physician's assistant did not acknowledge Ellen's presequence nor table it for a later time (i.e., "oh, okay, tell you what (.) let's come back to that in a few minutes during the examination so that I can check you out"). Instead, she implicitly dismisses Ellen's desire to talk about the cough, despite the fact that she went to the effort of referencing the nurse and emphasizing the significance of the problem—lasted 3 weeks and coughed up blood. As we argue in Chapters 3 and 4, this type of transition reflexively works to undermine the patient's ability to participate as a partner because of the asymmetry of the caregiver's choice to shift topics without addressing the patient's concern. The caregiver interactionally frames that issue as unimportant compared to the more salient topics that must now be advanced. As such, the move poses potential relational consequences as well as medical ones.

As the examination ensues, though, Ellen reveals that she has been taking cough syrup for the cough. Because Ellen is pregnant, the taking of medicine without the supervision of a health caregiver poses possible implications for the baby. As we observe in Chapter 3, when caregivers fail to follow up on issues that patients initiate, they risk slighting critical medical information, in this case, the patient's consumption of someone else's prescription cough syrup. If the physician's assistant did not intend to return to it later (and there is not interactional reason to believe that she planned to do so), Ellen could have continued engaging in unsafe health practices during pregnancy if she had not mentioned the taking of cough syrup later in the interaction.

In Excerpt 29, however, the physician's assistant tackles this problem. She does so through a combination of explanation and suggestive directives. Although the physician's assistant pursues this topic in a manner that avoids criticizing Ellen, the physician's assistant now confronts the challenge of recommending that Ellen shift from her present behavior to another one (i.e., from consuming such medicine to not doing so). Furthermore, she needs to educate Ellen about the dangers without jeopardizing aspects of Ellen's face. Although Ellen does not display any knowledge that taking someone else's prescription medicine is not appropriate (nor even legal) under any circumstance, especially pregnancy, nothing would be gained by overtly criticizing Ellen or by making her feel ignorant; she lacks confidence in the encounter already. To empower Ellen to participate as a partner, the physician's assistant has to help her understand the implications of her behavior and to make good choices for herself and for her unborn child. The physician's assistant offers an alternative health practice first (i.e., using honey as opposed to medicine) and then gives a more specific directive.

Excerpt 29:

```
 1   C:   >you've been< taking cough syrup (.) for that?
 2   P:   uh ya:h (.) I've (.) I took >some ov my huz< (.) exhusband's
 3        momz (.) prescription (.) cough syrup (.) cause >she had
 4        had< it (.)
 5   C:   mmuh huh (.1)
 6   P:   but (.) u:h (.) now it >seemed ta< (.) make my face swell
 7        up< (.) >an stuff< (.) >so I< quit taking that (.1)
 8   C:   okay (.2) the other thing that you >can do< (.) instead ov
 9        taking cough me:dicine=
10   P:   =mmhmm=
11   C:   iz >just take< some ho:ney (.) an mix some lemon juice
12        >in with it< (.)
13   P:   mm=
14   C:   =an take uh bit teaspoon >ov tha:t< (.)
15   P:   mm (.)
16   C:   >an that'll< sometimes coat (.) just so:oth that u:h (.)
17        irritated throat=
18   P:   =mm (.)
19   C:   >doesn't look< like >you've got< strep throat (.) cause
20        there's no puss on your tonsils (.) >an you're< not real
21        enlarged (.) itz >some mild< redness there=
22   P:   =mm=
23   C:   =but itz not >just uh< virus (.5) I'd like you not ta
24        take< too many medicines >when you're< pregnant (.3) at
25        least that's not necessary (.)
26   P:   yah (.6)
27   C:   iz >this uh< scar? (.)
28   P:   no (.) just >stretch marks<
```

Although the physician's assistant describes an alternative solution to Ellen's cough problem, she receives little input from Ellen with regard to whether or not Ellen understands nor what Ellen plans to do. Furthermore, despite the fact that posing the alternative suggests that something is wrong with taking medications during pregnancy and despite the assertion that "I'd like you not ta take too many medicines >when you're< pregnant," the physician's assistant still does not inform Ellen why she wants her to alter her behavior. Lacking such a rationale, Ellen may not perceive the importance of considering the honey and lemon juice alternative. The two let the topic drop in line 26 without a dialogue to facilitate interactive learning and without a full collaborative weighing of the options.

In Excerpt 30, the physician's assistant returns to the subject once more after an unrelated prior discussion. Although she offers Ellen one more option to consuming someone else's prescription medicine, the "why" portion of the entire conversation is missing, hence another abandoned "golden moment" for patient learning and for potential improvement in patient wellness.

Excerpt 30:

```
1   P:    kk kk (.2)
2   C:>   >if ya< want me to (.) I can >give you sa uh< mild cough
3         medicine (.) if >you think< that would help (.2) I'd
4         rather give it to ya (.) than >have you< take someone
5         else's=
6   P:    =ha ha=
7   C:    okay? (.1) >not uh< good ide:a to take >other people's<
8         medicine (.1) especially >if it's< prescribed=
9   P:    =mmhmm
```

Excerpt 30 illustrates the integration of directives as suggestions. The physician's assistant marks her appreciation for Ellen's knowledge of her body and her cough. She offers to give her a mild medication, extending the choice to Ellen—"if >you think< that would help." However, again, interactive learning constitutes an essential component of a collaborative, partnership orientation to health care encounters, and, in these three excerpts, the interactants do not share enough information for an interactive dialogue to transpire. Ellen reveals little about her preconceptions, beliefs, and thoughts; the physician's assistant provides Ellen with minimal information with which to make an intelligent, informed choice about future behavior, and Ellen stops short of pursuing that information, gaining that insight, using her caregiver as a resource.

Unlike the interaction between the caregiver and Margaret in Excerpt 25 in Chapter 4, dialogues do not tend to occur, leaving a void of ambiguity, uncertainty, and only tentative advancement toward the realization of collaboratively co-achieved educational and medical goals. Even when the caregiver offers explanations as in Excerpts 18 and 22, patients need to display their orientations to that information. Yet the paradox for patients comes when they combine this need, and perhaps desire, with other interactional asymmetries that occur during typical conversations with their caregivers (e.g., modernist, caregiver-initiated transitions and caregiver disconfirmation of patient presequences). Such asymmetries deter subsequent patient efforts to present themselves as partners when caregivers do not co-define them as such.

As we note in the previous chapters, however, caregivers also struggle with the both–and-ness of the logistical and medical necessity of attending to a number of issues in a short time frame as well as the relational, educational, and medical consequences of taking that lead in an abrupt manner. We suggest that caregivers and patients work together to co-produce the type of interactional framing that we discuss in Chapter 2. By co-orienting to the overlap and importance of topics (i.e., through joint contributions to the conversation—not caregiver monologues), caregivers and patients can collaboratively control the direction of the interaction. Through the mutual posing of and responding to issues as active listeners and co-participants, caregivers and patients simultaneously facilitate a conducive interactional and relational dynamic wherein interactive patient learning and a collaborative approach to medical procedures and preferred health practices may occur.

A REVIEW

As this chapter indicates, the co-accomplishment of medical goals depends on the reflexivity of relational and educational activities. In order for patients to become partners in their health care, they must be interactionally included in the co-achievement of medical tasks, from the taking of histories to the implementing of procedures. They must also be involved as a collaborator on the co-construction of possible solutions for medical concerns, employing their caregivers as resource people and expert guides.

However, for such a model to work, patients require information. They need to know what is going on during health care interactions and why. They need to participate in co-determining what issues become relevant and which fall by the wayside. They need to be given a voice as well as initiate a voice. Yet, as we have noted time and time again throughout this book, those voices rarely get lifted to ask questions, to seek answers, to probe for more information, to put forth their multiplicity of identities and goals. Further, this process must be reciprocal and collaborative. When both caregivers and patients pursue presequences (i.e., "This sounds important to you. What's up?") and ask confirmatory questions (i.e., "Tell me if this is what you mean . . ." or "What could we do to make this workable for you?"), they work toward a sharedness of understanding and a co-construction of mutually agreeable plans of action.

While the silence continues, though, examinations and procedures will go on; recommendations will be given; patients will come and go from health care facilities. Yet, it is no longer an issue of patients "just not complying" and caregivers "just not persuading." The postmodern era demands a dialogue, not as a nicety or some "relational thing," but as a medical necessity for more positive health outcomes for women.

Partnership for Health:
Continuing the Dialogue

I was in the midst of finishing this project when I popped part of my back out of place. As a sufferer of scoliosis, this happens to me quite a bit so I have a pretty high tolerance for the discomfort, especially when I am on a deadline. However, after about a week of trying to write with my back throbbing, I finally called my doctor for an appointment to have a back adjustment.

Although I really like my doctor (who is one of the faculty members at the osteopathic medical school at the university where I teach), I get impatient with how much time is spent in the waiting room as well as the time spent in the examining room between visits from the nurse and the doctor. On this particular occasion, however, I was taken into the examining room very quickly, and I was promptly visited by one of the nurses who took my vital signs and recorded my problem on the chart.

As usual, I pulled out my work from my bookbag to keep myself occupied while waiting for the doctor. However, I had just opened my folder when the door opened. A young woman entered the room, wearing a name tag that prominantly indicated her status as a first-year medical student. I smiled at her, but I groaned inside. I had been making super time, and this unexpected twist pretty much ensured a significant delay.

After about 10 minutes of patiently answering her questions (and getting increasingly frustrated because I knew that any really relevant questions would have to be repeated when my doctor arrived), I attempted to re-direct the conversation, to bring it to a quicker conclusion (similar to what I do when I'm talking with a very nice telemarketer with an unappealing product). "Ya know," I said to her, "at the moment, only my back bothers me. Ya see, the bone is sticking out of place right here." I pointed to the spot. The medical student then meticulously diagrammed my back on the chart. The clock continued to tick.

Finally, my doctor came into the room. We greeted each other, and the medical student gave her report. She settled back to observe our encounter, likely expecting the "usual," the "routine." However, my visits with this doctor do not fall into the modernist trap of simplistic and narrow conceptions of stereotypical caregiver–patient encounters, and, despite the increasing emphasis on patient-centered encounters in current medical school programs, I doubt that the medical student's prior conception of such encounters fit with the complexity of our emergent encounter. I find visits with my doctor to be extremely entertaining, valuable, and satisfying, in part because our interactions exemplify those of a postmodern relationship and of a partnership.

As we got started, he asked, "So, how's it going?" "Fine," I said. "No you're not, or you wouldn't be here," he noted. "You're right," I chuckled briefly, "I threw my back out about a week ago, and I'm working on this book and teaching in our off-campus master's program so I don't want to take the muscle relaxers that you gave to me because I can't fall asleep." "Even the Lodine?" he probed. "Well, I do always take it with the Flexoril so I'm not really sure. I just don't want to feel spacey," I answered. "That one's not supposed to do that, just stuff like the Flexoril," the doctor explained. "I'll try it," I said.

"So, where does it hurt?" he said, starting to feel my back. I pointed to the spot on my back. "Right there," I said, "Do you feel the bone?" He felt around my back. "Yup. You're tight across the shoulders too," he said, "all right, hop up on the table." As he prepared to adjust my back, we talked about attending the university's graduation ceremonies, and he inquired about my book and summer teaching schedule. I complained about being over-commited and battling time crunches. The doctor revealed that he had been away for some time and had to scramble to get a syllabus done. I told him I could identify.

He started working on one part of my back, told me that he was interested in a graduate program, and asked me about the one in my department. I gave him my opinion of a few of the other graduate programs at the university, and we laughed and talked about possibilities. He finally got to the most problematic part of my back. He popped it back into place, and I sat up. He asked me about a nonmedical-task personal difficulty with which I had been struggling for some time, and he teased me about my inability to just resolve the situation.

As I stood up and the doctor went to the desk in the room, I glanced at the medical student. She had a dazed expression on her face. I laughed and said, "Are you with us?" She said, "I've never seen doctors and patients talk with each other like that before." The doctor and I joined in joking with her that I was some sort of canned patient, just to give the medical students an example of a very different type of dynamic.

As he started to leave, he gave me a few final instructions, jokingly admonishing about my personal situation once more, and I offered him a couple of last words of wisdom about the graduate school issue. The medical student just followed him out of the room. Like us, she had just been through a whirlwind of attention to the multiplicity of fragmented identities that swirled around us and that we chose to momentarily grasp and highlight—fellow professionals, fellow scholars, fellow holders of graduate degrees, fellow educators, fellow parents, fellow frazzled people in an ever-changing, constantly hectic and chaotic world, fellow health care participants, fellow partners in my health care.

However, our encounter lasted only around 12 minutes, only 2 minutes more than the monolithic, one-dimensional question–answer session that I had with the medical student. Through the nature of our interaction, we co-oriented to our vast array of identities, goals, and perspectives as interdependent, not separate; as reflexive, not distant. Our collaboratively co-constructed interactional framing enabled us to attend to "the business at hand" (my back) while simultaneously and reflexively responding to many of the other lurking identities and issues that we chose not to treat as irrelevant or nonconsequential. By dabbling more than dwelling, by affirming more than disconfirming, we co-achieved an expedient encounter that fit within the chaotic, frantic pace of our respective lives, thus again, reflexively reaffirming parts of our identities and goals.

Like the interactions between the nursing student and the female doctor in Chapter 2 and between the university professor and the female doctor in Chapter 3, this type of relational dynamic may be an anomaly; not all caregivers and patients share so many commonalities in addition to their identities as "caregiver" and "patient." Furthermore, they may restrict themselves with what they choose to make relevant during the examination and limit themselves with regard to the complexity and potential multidimensional nature of the emergent relational dynamic. Yet, we would contend that all co-created relationships between caregivers and patients emerge as intricate, unique entities; like snowflakes, they may be made out of the same substance, but they never quite take the same shape. Unlike snowflakes, however, each relationship embodies a plethora of potentially diverse and often conflicting configurations, even those wherein the interactants focus on medical problems. The nature of human beings in this era makes unidimensional relational and individual definitions naïve oversimplifications.

In this book, we have pursued relationships between caregivers and patients in light of the postmodern condition, appreciating and embracing the complexities, the fragmentation, the inconsistencies, the frenzy, the temporality, the ambiguity, and perhaps most important, the reflexivity of contemporary relationships. Our goal has not been to provide "answers"; indeed, such a focus would contradict the essence of the project. Instead, we have strived to offer a catalyst for continued dialogues about health care encounters between members of the medical and academic communities and between people, especially women, for whom these encounters are particularly consequential. As a means of summarizing the arguments that were outlined in this volume, we highlight what we consider to be the primary contributions of this work, and we then advance important research questions for future analysis of health care encounters from this postmodern perspective.

PRIMARY CONTRIBUTIONS

As we started this project, we were particularly excited about our opportunity to share our collection of data from a variety of women's health care interactions. We wanted to contribute to the ongoing effort to understand health care interactions by looking at naturally occurring interactions and by focusing on the co-construction of those interactions by the participants. As we look back over this project, we certainly feel pleased with our ability to provide exemplars of such interactions, and we feel that those examples of naturally occurring interaction between caregivers and patients can serve as a catalyst for understanding and for contemplating what transpires between caregivers and patients.

Yet, in addition to this book's empirical contribution to the medical and academic communities, we feel that this book also enriches the body of knowledge theoretically. Although we genuinely hope that caregivers and patients find the information in this volume useful and even inspiring as they take our descriptions and contentions into their own health care encounters, we believe that this book extends beyond a how-to book. We contend that health care encounters constitute interactional events that preclude "tips" which all can employ to make their encounters "better." As such, we have strived to provide theoretical explanations that underlie our suggestions, stressing a way of thinking about health care encounters—not simply ways of engaging in health care exchanges.

Postmodern Perspective of Health Care Encounters

We began this project with the objective of offering an understanding of the complexities of interpersonal communication in the health care context. Although our earlier work clearly illustrates that we did not quite begin this venture as postmodernists (if we may be so bold as to give ourselves a monolithic label at this point), we come to the close of this part of our journey clutching at pieces of road signs that keep pointing in the direction of postmodernism.

When we examine the splintering of our society and the swirling of mixed messages, conflicting data, and scrambled ideas, we realize that no certainty may exist except that there is no certainty, only fragmented perspectives. Hence, simplistic efforts to produce monolithic descriptions, whether by scholars or individuals who stumble through the maze of everyday life, must end in frustration. Despite our best attempts to talk through the complexities in this volume, the linearity of writing condemns us to inadequacy; we always fall short of capturing anything, much less something as inherently dynamic and emergent as human relationships.

However, in terms of understanding health care encounters, we suggest that this postmodern perspective enables us to embrace, not ignore, the complexity of such interactions wherein fragmented relational and individual identities, goals, preconceptions, and perspectives intersect. Furthermore, this postmodern orientation permits us to probe the paradoxes, acknowledging the simultaneous and potentially conflicting nature of those identities, goals, preconceptions, and perspectives. On many occasions during the writing of this book, we found ourselves shaking our heads, pondering the seemingly irreconcilableness of perpetual both–and-ness, wondering how incongruent identities and incompatible goals may co-exist, yet realizing that none can just be cast away or aside without consequence (relationally, educationally, medically).

The struggle in everyday life ensues as interactants in interpersonal communication situations (not simply health care interactions) strive to reconcile the both–and-ness. Yet, in so doing, they find themselves in multiple concurrent mazes, stumbling through openings in one while crashing into a brick wall in another simultaneously. As we have noted recurrently throughout this book, such paradoxes can be consequential for the co-accomplishment of relational, educational, and medical goals.

Advancement of Relational Communication Theory

By taking this postmodern perspective of interpersonal communication in the health care context, we necessarily re-visited our understanding of writings in the area of relational communication. From the outset, we wanted to treat health care interactions as systems and to focus on the interdependence of health care participants; however, as our work here ensued, we came to appreciate that constantly emerging relationships do not simply move from one definition to another. Instead, interactants may co-construct a multiplicity of relational and individual definitions and co-orientations to each other and the encounter. As such, we strive in this volume to employ the premises of relational communication theory in our postmodern approach to health care encounters, yet we do not do so monolithically—in terms of potentiality of relational definitions nor in terms of aspects of relational communication (i.e., a strict focus on "control").

Although previous work in the area of relational communication refers to interactional paradoxes, we build on those works to discuss relational paradoxes for health caregivers and patients that is consistent with postmodernism. Because of inherent confusion, amidst idealistic preferences for clarity, because individuals in this era confront uncertainties with regard to expectations, because knowledge must be treated as temporal, emergent, and potentially conflicting, and because of the multiplicity of identities and goals, caregivers and patients struggle with both–and like relational paradoxes. More than ever before, identities interwine, and modernist-like efforts at denying all but one identity or reality force ever-changing, ever-emergent individuals and relationships into tight, static pigeon holes.

In this book, we explore the consequentiality of these relational paradoxes. We pursue how caregivers and patients display and treat concurrent relational and individual identities, and we note the face needs that emanate from emergent paradoxes of identity. As such, we offer a depiction of the complexities of relational communication within the women's health care setting, and we lay the groundwork for future research in the areas of relational paradoxes and relational communication from a postmodern perspective.

Reflexivity of Goals

Even in our own previous work on multiple goals in the health care context, we treated goals in a primarily separate manner. However, our postmodern perspective prompted us to re-examine the complexity of goals, and our view of relational communication contributed to our re-thinking of the intertangled nature of those goals. This book offers a description of goals that embraces that complexity and interdependence and that delineates the reflexivity of interactional activities as well as the reflexivity of simultaneous relational, educational, and medical goals.

By examining health care interactions in light of the reflexivity of goals, we note the essentiality of relational activities for the co-accomplishment of educational and medical goals as well as the salience of how educational and medical goals get pursued for the co-attainment of important relational goals and activities. Throughout our descriptions of the exemplars in this book, we stress the consequentiality of the reflexivity of goals, especially in terms of the co-achievement of interactive learning and of a collaborative co-orientation to attaining mutually acceptable medical outcomes.

CONTINUING THE DIALOGUE
ON WOMEN'S HEALTH COMMUNICATION

As we conclude this book, countless women will visit their health caregivers. Their encounters will consist of a wide range of possible concerns, from preventative health care practices and procedures to sinus infections, from eye examinations to dental examinations to gynecologic examinations, from treatment for the flu to screening for HIV/AIDS or sexually transmitted diseases, from physical therapy for automobile accident victims to chemotherapy for cancer patients. These women enter examining rooms or treatment areas as only one aspect of their hectic, frazzled lives, yet their health, their wellness, impacts (and is a vital part of) all of those other facets of their lived realities.

If we leave our readers with only one thought, we would hope that it would be this: What happens during women's health care encounters *matters*; all verbal and nonverbal behaviors are consequential for the collaborative co-definition of the encounter, for their individual and relational identities, for the ways in which multiple relational, educational, and medical goals are advanced or hindered. For the brief moment in time that caregivers and patients come together, they actively co-construct the emergent relational dynamic, and importantly, that relational dynamic must not be construed as insignificant simply because the interaction does not occur between friends, co-workers, or family members; it must not be viewed as some "nicety" that has little bearing on the "real" tasks at hand. The nature of the complex, multifaceted relational dynamic reflexively enables or hinders the concurrent co-attainment of educational and medical goals. As we have suggested throughout this book, the reflexivity of those activities and goals can work to facilitate or stifle interactive patient learning as well as a partnership-like co-orientation to acceptable health care practices.

We encourage others to pursue health care interactions, especially with women patients, from a postmodern perspective. In particular, we urge caregivers and patients to attend interactionally to the multiplicity and complexity of their identities and goals. By maintaining a monolithic focus, both interactants risk missing those "golden moments" where learning and where collaboration can occur with critical possible health consequences.

We also harken to our academic colleagues to conduct more research that examines the post-encounter implications of talk that recognizes the postmodern condition as well as interactions that remain wed to the constraints of a modernist treatment of roles, education, and recommendations. Notably, this orientation to health care encounters extends beyond, yet includes, the now vogue "patient-centered" efforts. Yet, as we advance these arguments for an even more interactive, collaborative, partnership-like dynamic, we recognize the need for empirical studies that pursue our assertions about the value of such an intuitively sound position.

Despite the constant need for more information on women's health care encounters, we close now by reiterating that no body of research can ever be complete and that our collective and individual understandings will never be "whole" or "finished," based on some external absolute "fact." As such, we emphasize that the lack of certainty that prevails in the postmodern era perpetuates and reifies the need for dialogues to continue. Of course, those conversations must occur between members of academic and medical education communities, but the most important dialogues must take place between caregivers and patients.

Our final plea is that caregivers and patients will embrace—not shun—the complexity of the postmodern condition, affirming their diverse identities, empowering patients to become partners in their own health care through interactive learning and collaborative co-constructions of acceptable health practices. Only as caregivers and patients slice through silence with the powerful sword of conversation can they co-accomplish conducive relational dynamics for partnerships that aggressively battle threats to the wellness of women, especially those stemming from the ignorance or passivity of either caregivers or patients.

Appendix A:
Description of Data

University Health Care Facility

The researchers (Sandra L. Ragan and Michael Pagano) obtained the permission of a female nurse practitioner at a large southwestern university's health care facility for the recording of conversations between her and her patients. All women patients were asked to review a description of the study and to give their verbal consents for their voices to be recorded. (The university's Institutional Review Board mandated verbal rather than written consent to ensure patient anonymity.)

The patients were primarily university students who were seeking contraception and/or gynecologic examinations. The participants ranged in age from 18 to 33 years old. Of the 60 patients who visited the nurse practitioner during the period of data collection, 56 (93%) agreed to participate in the study. However, a mechanical error occurred during 15 of those interactions, thus the available data from this research effort consists of 41 audiotaped interactions between the female nurse practitioner and her patients.

These interactions were transcribed by the researchers. First, the interactions were transcribed verbatim. To capture the micro-details of the talk (i.e., in terms of pauses, vocal hesitations, disfluencies, overlaps, etc.), we transcribed some of the excerpts in more detail by using the transcription notation system developed by Gail Jefferson (see Atkinson & Heritage, 1984, as well as Appendix B).

Native-American Health Care Facility

As part of her ethnographic study for her doctoral dissertation (under the direction of Sandra L. Ragan), Glenn (1990) obtained audiotaped recordings of interactions between caregivers and patients at an urban Native-American health care facility funded by the Indian Health Service, the Oklahoma Department of Human Services, the Bureau of Indian Affairs, and other nonprofit organizations. For the purposes of this book and some of our previous work, we use 26 audiotaped interactions between caregivers and their patients. The patients primarily came to the facility for prenatal care, and their caregivers were female, Euro-American nurses and a female, Euro-American physician's assistant.

Written consent was given by all participants after they had an opportunity to read a written description of the study. The audiotaped interactions were transcribed by the researchers in the same manner as the data set from the university health care facility.

Doctor's Office

The researcher (Athena DuPre) obtained the permission of a Euro-American, female medical doctor to gather ethnographic and audiotaped data at her private practice office in a major southwestern city. This doctor was in her early 30s at the time of data collection, and she had been practicing medicine for approximately 3 years. Her medical training had included some communication training in which she engaged in practice interactions with patients and attained suggestions from mock patients and medical school faculty about her communication skills.

A family practice physician, she primarily examines Euro-American women and children who tend to be insured and who are in middle or upper class. During the time of data collection, her patients ranged in age from 2 weeks to 69 years. After reading a written description of the study, 53 patients agreed to participate in it by giving verbal consent, per the Institutional Review Board's approval of the study. (Only 3 other patients did not consent.)

DuPre took fieldnotes and recorded conversations with a hand-held recorder during each of these interactions. The typed fieldnotes and transcriptions of interactions serve as the data from this particular research project.

Ethnographies of Two Hospitals

Two researchers (Cynthia Wilkins and Christina S. Beck) obtained permission to conduct ethnographic research at two hospitals in a midwestern city. These hospitals were undergoing the initial stages of a "joint venture." One of the hospitals is a Catholic facility that is sponsored by an order of nuns, and the other is a privately owned, for-profit hospital. Although Wilkins (1996) detailed the implications of the two very diverse, organizational cultures on the emergent pre-merger and merger process in her doctoral dissertation (under the direction of Christina S. Beck), portions of the ethnographic fieldnotes were used in the present work to offer descriptive examples of caregiver–patient interaction in a hospital context.

Observations occurred during meetings between executives at the two hospitals as well as meetings between various department members and during shift changes in nursing units. Beck and Wilkins also shadowed doctors and nurses in both hospitals in various units, including the surgical unit, the outpatient surgery unit, the pediatric unit, the OB-GYN unit, and the emergency room. The research that involves caregiver–patient interactions took place over a 3-month period in late 1994 to early 1995, within the context of the larger study that transpired over a period of more than 1 year.

Appendix B:
Summary of Transcription Notations

The notations listed here include those that appear recurrently throughout the text. For a more extended description of conversation analytic notation symbols, please see Atkinson and Heritage (1984).

:	elongation of sound
> <	quickening of pace
BBBB	louder sound
(.)	vocal hesitation
(.2)	pause
bbb	stress on a particular sound
[ ]	overlap

References

Aaronson, K. D., Schwartz, J. S., Goin, J. E., & Mancini, D. M. (1995). Sex differences in patient acceptance of cardiac transplant candidacy. *Circulation, 91,* 2753–2761.

Alexander, K., & McCullough, J. (1981). Women's preferences for gynecological examiners: Sex versus role. *Women and Health, 6*(3/4), 123-134.

Allen, D., Gilchrist, V., Levinson, W., & Roter, D. (1993, November 15). Caring for women: Is it different? *Patient Care,* pp. 183–199.

Altman, L. K. (1991, August 6). Men, women and heart disease: More than a question of sexism. *The New York Times,* p. C1.

American Cancer Society. (1990). 1989 survey of physicians' attitudes and practices in early cancer detection. *CA-A Cancer Journal for Clinicians, 40,* 77–101.

American College of Obstetricians and Gynecologists. (1993, October 29). *Poll shows women rely on OB-GYNs for primary care* (news release). Washington, DC: Author.

American College of Obstetricians and Gynecologists. (1996, April 29). *New research on domestic violence and pregnancy outcomes* (news release). Washington, DC: Author.

Apple, R. (1990). *Women, health, and medicine in America: A historical handbook.* New York: Garland.

Arney, W., & Bergen, B. (1983). The chronic patient. *Sociology of Health and Illness, 5*(1), 1–4.

Arntson, P. (1985). Future research in health communication. *Journal of Applied Communication Research, 13*(2), 118–130.

Arntson, P. (1989). Improving citizens' health competencies. *Health Communication, 1*(1), 29–34.

Aronsson, K., & Satterlund-Larsson, U. (1987). Politeness strategies and doctor-patient communication: On the social choreography of collaborative thinking. *Journal of Language and Social Psychology, 6*(1), 1–27.

Atkinson, J., & Heritage, J. (Eds.). (1984). *Structures of social action: Studies in conversational analysis.* Cambridge: Cambridge University Press.

Austoker, J., & Sharp, D. (1993). Breast cancer and benign breast disease. In A. McPherson (Ed.), *Women's problems in general practice* (3rd ed., pp. 16–49). Oxford: Oxford University Press.

Ballard-Reisch, D. S. (1990). A model of participative decision making for physician–patient interaction. *Health Communication, 2*(2), 91–104.

Ballard-Reisch, D. (1993). Health care providers and consumers: Making decisions together. In B. C. Thornton & G. L. Kreps (Eds.), *Perspectives on health communication* (pp. 66–80). Prospect Heights, IL: Waveland Press.

Barrett, M., & Roberts, H. (1978). Doctors and their patients: The social control of women in general practice. In C. Smart & B. Smart (Eds.), *Women, sexuality and social control* (pp. 41–52). London: Routledge & Kegan Paul.

Bateson, G. (1935). Culture contact and schismogenisis. *Man, 35,* 178–183.

Bateson, G. (1951). Information and codification: A philosophical approach. In J. Ruesch & G. Bateson (Eds.), *Communication: The social matrix of psychiatry* (pp. 168–211). New York: Norton.

Bateson, G. (1955). A theory of play and fantasy. *Psychiatric Research Reports, II,* 39–51.

Bateson, G. (1958). *Naven.* Stanford: Stanford University Press.

Bateson, G. (1972). *Steps to an ecology of mind.* New York: Ballantine.

Bateson, G. (1979). *Mind and nature: A necessary unit.* New York: Dutton.

Batt, S. (1994). *Patient no more: The politics of breast cancer.* Charlottetown, PEI, Canada: Guneray Books.

Bavelas, J. B. (1991). Some problems with linking goals to discourse. In K. Tracy (Ed.), *Understanding face-to-face interaction: Issues linking goals and discourse* (pp. 119–130). Hillsdale, NJ: Lawrence Erlbaum Associates.

Baxter, L. (1984). Trajectories of relationship disengagement. *Journal of Social and Personal Relationships, 1,* 29–48.

Baxter, L., & Montgomery, B. (1996). *Relating dialogues and dialectics.* New York: Guilford.

Beach, W. A. (1995). Preserving and constraining options: "Okays" and "official" priorities in medical interviews. In G. H. Morris & R. J. Chenail (Eds.), *The talk of the clinic: Explorations in the analysis of medical and therapeutic discourse* (pp. 259–290). Hillsdale, NJ: Lawrence Erlbaum Associates.

Beck, C. (1994). How can I tell you this?: The interactional nature of narratives. *Journal of the Northwest Communication Association, 22,* 5–26.

Beck, C. (1995). You make the call: The co-creation of media text through interaction in an interpretive community of Giant fans. *La Revue de Electronique (the Electronic Journal of Communication), 5.*

Beck, C. (1996). "I've got some points I'd like to make here": The achievement of social face through turn management during the 1992 vice-presidential debate. *Political Communication, 13*(2), 165–180.

Beck, C., & Aden, R. (1996). *"Huh, huh, huh, cool": Beavis and Butt-head: The process of interpretive community formation and the postmodern paradox.* Unpublished manuscript.

Beck, C., & Ragan, S. (1992). Negotiating relational and medical talk: Frame shifts in the gynecologic exam. *Journal of Language and Social Psychology, 11*(1), 47–61.

Beck, C., & Ragan, S. (1995). The impact of relational activities on the accomplishment of practitioner and patient goals in the gynecologic examination. In G. Kreps & D. O'Hair (Eds.), *Communication and health outcomes* (pp. 73–86). Cresskill, NJ: Hampton Press.

Beck, C., & Wilkins, C. (1996). *The continual struggle to define culture in ever changing organizations: The clash of two cultural values in a pre-"joint venture" hospital.* Unpublished manuscript.

Becker, R., Terrin, M., Ross, R., Knatterud, G., Desvigne-Nickens, P., Gore, J., Braunwald, E., & the Thromboloysis Myocardial Infarction Investigators. (1994). Comparison clinical outcomes for women and men after acute myocardial infarction. *Annals of Internal Medicine,* 638–645.

Beisecker, A. E., & Beisecker, T. D. (1990). Patient information-seeking behaviors when communicating with doctors. *Medical Care, 28*(1), 19–28.

Bell, N. (1992). Women and AIDS: Too little, too late. In H. Holmes & L. Purdy (Eds.), *Feminist perspectives in medical ethics* (pp. 83–92). Bloomington: Indiana University Press.

Bensing, J. M., Brink-Muinen, A., & DeBakker, D. (1993). Gender differences in practice style: A Dutch study of general practitioners. *Medical Care, 31*(3), 219–29.

Bennett, J. C. (1993). Inclusion of women in clinical trials—Policies for population subgroups. *New England Journal of Medicine, 329*, 288–292.

Berger, P., & Luckmann, T. (1966). *The social construction of reality: A treatise in the sociology of knowledge*. Garden City, NY: Doubleday.

Bermosk, L. S., & Porter, S. E. (1979). *Women's health and human wholeness*. New York: Appleton-Century-Crofts.

Bille, D. A. (Ed.). (1981). *Practical approaches to patient teaching*. Boston: Little, Brown.

Billings, J., & Stoeckle, J. (1977). Pelvic examination instruction and the doctor-patient relationship. *Journal of Medical Education, 52*, 834–839.

Boden, D. (1994). *The business of talk organizations in action*. Cambridge, MA: Blackwell.

Boden, D., & Zimmerman, D. H. (Eds.). (1991). *Talk and social structure: Studies in ethnomethodology and conversation analysis*. Berkeley: University of California Press.

Brink-Muinen, A., DeBakker, D., & Bensing, J. (1994). Consultations for women's health problems: Factors influencing women's choice of sex of general practitioner. *British Journal of General Practice, 44*, 205-210.

Brody, J. E. (1994, January 8). Little good news on Americans' health habits. *The New York Times*, p. C:12.

Brody, J. E. (1995, March 8). Personal health. *The New York Times*, p. C12.

Brown, P., & Levinson, S. C. (1987). *Politeness: Some universals in language use*. Cambridge, England: Cambridge University Press.

Budoff, P. (1994). Women's centers: A model for future health cares. In J. Sechzer, A. Griffin, & S. Pfallin (Eds.), *Forging a women's health research agenda: Policy issues for the 1990's* (pp. 165–170). New York: The New York Academy of Science.

Buller, M., & Buller, D. B. (1987). Physicians, communication style and patient satisfaction. *Journal of Health and Social Science, 28*, 375–388.

Burgoon, J., Pfau, M., Parrott, R., Birk, T., Coker, R., & Burgoon, M. (1987). Relational communication, satisfaction, compliance-gaining strategies, and compliance in communication between physicians and patients. *Communication Monographs, 54*, 307–324.

Burgoon, M., Birk, T. S., & Hall, J. R. (1991). Compliance and satisfaction with physician-patient communication: An expectancy theory interpretation of gender differences. *Human Communication Research, 18*, 177–208.

Burgoon, M., Parrott, R., Burgoon, J., Coker, R., Pfau, M., & Birk, T. (1990). Patients' severity of illness, noncompliance, and locus for control and physicians' compliance-gaining messages. *Health Communication, 2*, 29–46.

Burke, K. (1950). *A rhetoric of motives*. Los Angeles: University of California Press.

Calnan, M. (1984). Clinical uncertainty: Is it a problem in the doctor-patient relationship? *Sociology of Health and Illness, 6*(1), 74–85.

Cardello, L. L., Ray, E. B., & Pettey, G. R. (1995). The relationship of perceived physician communicator style to patient satisfaction. *Communication Reports, 8*(1), 27-37.

Charo, R. A. (1993). Protecting us to death: Women pregnancy and clinical research trials. *Saint Louis University Law Journal, 38*, 135–187.

Chenail, R. (Ed.). (1991). *Medical discourse and systemic frames of comprehension*. Norwood, NJ: Ablex.

Cheney, G. (1983). The rhetoric of identification and the study of organizational communication. *Quarterly Journal of Speech, 69*, 143–58.

Cicourel, A. V. (1968). *The social organization of juvenile justice*. New York: Wiley.

Cicourel, A. V. (1970). Basis and normative rules in the negotiation of status and role. In H. P. Dreitzel (Ed.), *Recent sociology* (Vol. 2, pp. 4–45). New York: Macmillan.

Cicourel, A. V. (1980). Three models of discourse analysis: The role of social structure. *Discourse Process, 3,* 101–132.

Cichon, E. J., & Masterson, J. T. (1993). Physician-patient communication: Mutual role expectations. *Communication Quarterly, 41*(4), 477–489.

Cissna, K. N., & Sieburg, E. (1981). Patterns of interactional confirmation and disconfirmation. In C. Wilder-Mott & J. H. Weakland (Eds.), *Rigor and imagination: Essays from the legacy of Gregory Bateson* (pp. 253–282). New York: Praeger.

Clancy, C. M., & Massion, C. T. (1992). American women's health: A patchwork quilt with gaps. *Journal of the American Medical Association, 268,* 1918–1919.

Clark, J. A., & Mishler, E. G. (1992). Attending to patients' stories: Reframing the clinical task. *Sociology of Health and Illness, 14*(3), 344–372.

Clarke, K. W., Gray, D., Keating, N. A., & Hampton, J. R. (1994). Do women with acute myocardial infarction receive the same treatment as men? *British Medical Journal, 309,* 563–565.

Cohen, S. J., Halvorson, H. W., & Gosselink, C. A. (1994). Changing physical behavior to improve disease prevention. *Preventative Medicine, 23,* 284–291.

Colditz, G. (1990, July/August). The nurses' health study: Findings during 10 years of follow up of a cohort of U.S. women. *Current Problems in Obstetrics, Gynecology and Fertility,* 131–172.

Coleman, W. (1983). The struggle for control in health care settings: Political implications of language use. *Et cetera, 40,* 401–408.

Collins, R. (1981a). Micro-translations as a theory-building strategy. In K. Knorr-Cetina & A. V. Cicourel (Eds.), *Advances in social theory and methodology: Toward an integration of micro- and macro-sociologies* (pp. 81–108). Boston: Routledge & Kegan Paul.

Collins, R. (1981b). On the microfoundation of macrosociology. *American Journal of Sociology, 86,* 964–1014.

Collins, R. (1987). Interaction ritual chains, power and property: The micro–macro connection as an empirically based problem. In J. C. Alexander, B. Giesen, R. Munch, & N. J. Smelser (Eds.), *The micro–macro link* (pp. 193–206). Berkeley: University of California.

The Commonwealth Fund. (1993). *The commonwealth fund survey of women's health.* New York: Author.

Corea, G. (1977). *The hidden malpractice: How American medicine treats women as patients and professionals.* New York: William Morrow.

Coulthard, M., & Ashby, M. (1976). A linguistic description of doctor–patient interview. In M. Wadsworth & D. Robinson (Eds.), *Studies in everyday medical life* (pp. 69–88). London: Martin Robertson.

Council on Ethical and Judicial Affairs. (1991). Gender disparities in clinical decision making. *Journal of the American Medical Association, 266,* 559–562.

Courtright, J., Millar, F., & Rogers, L. (1983). A new measure of interaction control patterns. *Communication, 12,* 47–68.

Coyne, J. C. (1985). Toward a theory of frames and reframing: The social nature of frames. *Journal of Marital and Family Therapy, 11*(4), 337–344.

Crable, R. (1977). Ike: Identification, argument, and paradoxical appeal. *Quarterly Journal of Speech, 63,* 188–195.

Craig, R. T., Tracy, K., & Spisak, F. (1986). The discourse of requests: Assessment of a politeness approach. *Human Communication Research, 12,* 437–468.

Crook, M. (1995). *My body: Women speak out about their health care.* New York: Insight Books.

Cupach, W. R., & Metts, S. (1994). *Facework.* Thousand Oaks, CA: Sage.

Davies, P. (1981). Categorisation, framing and the structuring of psychiatric assessment. In P. Atkinson & C. Heath (Eds.), *Medical Work* (pp. 19–40). Farnborough, Hampshire, England: Gower.

Davis, M. S. (1968). Variations in patients' compliance with doctors' advice: An empirical analysis of patterns of communication. *American Journal of Public Health, 58*(2), 274–88.

Davis, K. (1985). Story-telling and the exercise of the power. In T. Hak, J. Haafkens, & G. Nijof (Eds.), *Working papers on discourse and conversational analysis* (pp. 107–120). Rotterdam, Denmark: Erasmus Universiteit Rotterdam, Instituut voor Preventieve en Sociale Psychiatrie.

Davis, K. (1988a). Paternalism under the microscope. In A. D. Todd & S. Fisher (Eds.), *Gender and discourse: The power of talk* (pp. 19–54). Norwood, NJ: Ablex.

Davis, K. (1988b). *Power under the microscope.* Dordrecht, The Netherlands: Foris.

Davis, K. (1993). Cultural dopes and she-devils: Cosmetic surgery as ideological dilemma. In K. Davis & S. Fisher (Eds.), *Negotiating at the margins: The gendered discourses of power and resistance* (pp. 23–47). New Brunswick, NJ: Rutgers University Press.

Davis, K., & Fisher, S. (Eds.). (1993). *Negotiating at the margins: The gendered discourses of power and resistance.* New Brunswick, NJ: Rutgers University Press.

Domar, A. (1985–1986). Psychological aspects of the pelvic exam: Individual needs and physician involvement. *Women and Health, 10,* 75–90.

Drass, K. E. (1988). Discourse and occupational perspective: A comparison of nurse practitioners and physician assistants. *Discourse Processes, 11,* 163–181.

Drew, P., & Heritage, J. (Eds.). (1992). *Talk at work.* Cambridge: Cambridge University Press.

DuPre, A. A., & Beck, C. (in press). "How can I put this?" Exaggerated self-disparagement as alignment strategy during problematic disclosures by patients to doctors. *Qualitative Health Research.*

Duck, S. (1992). *Human relations.* Newbury Park, CA: Sage.

Duncan, H. (1967). The search for a social theory of communication in American sociology. In F. Dance (Ed.), *Human communication theory* (pp. 236–263). New York: Holt, Rinehart & Winston.

Eaker, E., Chesebro, J. H., Sacks, F. M., Wenger, N. K., Whisnant, J. P., & Winston, M. (1993). Cardiovascular disease in women. *Circulation, 88,* 1999–2009.

Edelmann, R. J. (1994). Embarrassment and blushing: Factors influencing face-saving strategies. In S. Ting-Toomey (Ed.), *The challenge of facework* (pp. 231–268). Albany: State University of New York Press.

Elstad, J. (1994). Women's priorities regarding physician behavior and their preference for a female physician. *Women and Health, 21*(4), 1–19.

Emerson, J. (1970). Behavior in private places: Sustaining definitions of reality in gynecological examinations. In H. P. Dreitzel (Ed.), *Recent sociology, No. 2: Patterns of communicative behavior* (pp. 73–97). New York: Macmillan.

Emmert, V. J. L. (1989). Interaction analysis. In P. Emmert & L. L. Barker (Eds.), *Measurement of communicative behavior* (pp. 218–248). New York: Longman.

Eraker, S. A., Kirscht, J. P., & Becker, M. H. (1984). Understanding and improving patient compliance. *Annals of Internal Medicine, 100,* 258–268.

Ericson, P. M., & Rogers, L. (1973). New procedures for analyzing relational communication. *Family Process, 12*(3), 245–267.

Ervin-Tripp, S. M. (1971). Sociolinguistics. In J. A. Fishman (Ed.), *Advances in the sociology of language* (pp. 15–91). The Hague: Mouton.

Evans, D. A., Block, M. R., Steinberg, E. R., & Penrose, A. M. (1986). Frames and heuristics in doctor-patient discourse. *Social Science Medicine, 22*(10), 1027–1034.

Fang, W., Hillard, P., Lindsay, R., & Underwood, P. (1984). Evaluation of students' clinical and communication skills in performing a gynecologic examination. *Journal of Medical Education, 59,* 758–760.

Falvo, D. R. (1985). *Effective patient education: A guide to increase compliance.* Rockville, MD: Aspen.

Federman, D. D. (1990). The education of medical students: Sounds, alarms, and excursions. *Academic Medicine, 65,* 221–226.

Fee, E. (Ed.). (1982). *Women and health: The politics of sex in medicine.* Farmingdale, NY: Baywood.

Finck, K. (1986). The potential health care crisis of hysterectomy. In D. Kjernik & I. Martinson (Eds.), *Women in health and illness: Life experience and crisis* (pp. 200–217). Philadelphia, PA: Saunders.

Fisher, S. (1984). Doctor-patient communication: A social and micro-political performance. *Sociology of Health and Illness, 6,* 1–29.

Fisher, S. (1986). *In the patients' best interests: Women and the politics of medical decisions.* New Brunswick, NJ: Rutgers University Press.

Fisher, S. (1991). A discourse of the social: Medical talk/power talk/oppositional talk. *Discourse and Society, 2*(2), 157–182.

Fisher, S. (1993a). Gender, power, resistance: Is care the remedy? In K. Davis & S. Fisher (Eds.), *Negotiating at the margins: The gendered discourses of power and resistance* (pp. 87–121). New Brunswick, NJ: Rutgers University Press.

Fisher, S. (1993b). Doctor talk/patient talk: How treatment decisions are negotiated in doctor-patient communication. In A. Todd & S. Fisher (Eds.), *The social organization of doctor-patient communication* (pp. 161–182). Norwood, NJ: Ablex.

Fisher, S. (1995). *Nursing wounds: Nurse practitioners/doctors/women patients/and the negotiation of meaning.* New Brunswick, NJ: Rutgers University Press.

Fisher, S., & Groce, S. (1985). Doctor–patient negotiation of cultural assumptions. *Sociology of Health and Illness, 7,* 342–374.

Fisher, S., & Groce, S. (1990). Accounting practices in medical interviews. *Language in Society, 19,* 225–250.

Folger, J., & Poole, M. S. (1982). Relational coding schemes: The question of validity. In M. Burgoon (Ed.), *Communication yearbook 5* (pp. 235–247). New Brunswick, NJ: Transaction.

Foucault, M. (1979). *Discipline and punish.* New York: Random House.

Fox, S. A., Siu, A. L., & Stein, J. A. (1994). The importance of physician communication on breast cancer screening of older women. *Archives of Internal Medicine, 154,* 2058–2068.

Francis, J., & Wales, R. (1994). Speech a'la mode prosodic cues, message, interpretation, and impression formation. *Journal of Language and Social Psychology, 13*(1), 34–44.

Frankel, R. M. (1984). From sentence to sequence: Understanding the medical encounter through microinteractional analysis. *Discourse Processes, 7,* 135–170.

Frankel, R. M. (1989). I waz wondering—uhm could Raid uhm effect the brain permanently doya know?: Some observations on the intersection between speaking and writing in calls to a poison control center. *Western Journal of Speech Communication, 53*(2), 195–226.

Frankel, R. M. (1990). Talking in interviews: A dispreference for patient-initiated questions in physician–patient encounters. In G. Psathas (Ed.), *Interactional competence* (pp. 231–262). Washington, DC: University Press of America.

Frankel, R. M. (1993). The laying on of hands: Aspects of the organization of gaze, touch, and talk in a medical encounter. In A. D. Todd & S. Fisher (Eds.), *The social organization of doctor–patient communication* (pp. 71–106). Norwood, NJ: Ablex.

Frankel, R. M. (1995). Some answers about questions in clinical interviews. In G. H. Morris & R. J. Chenail (Eds.), *The talk of the clinic* (pp. 233–258). Hillsdale, NJ: Lawrence Erlbaum Associates.

Frankel, R. M., & Beckman, H. B. (1989). Conversation and compliance with treatment recommendations: An application of micro-interactional analysis in medicine. In L. Grossberg, B. J. O'Keefe, & E. Wartella (Eds.), *Rethinking communication* (Vol 2. pp. 60–74). London: Sage.

Friedman, E. (Ed.). (1994). *An unfinished revolution: Women and health care in America.* New York: United Hospital Fund of New York.

Gadamer, H. (1975). *Truth and method.* New York: Seabury.

Gadamer, H. (1976). *Philosophical hermeneutics.* Berkeley: University of California Press.

Gadamer, H. (1988). On the circle of understanding. In J. M. Connolly & T. Keutner (Eds.). *Hermeneutics versus science: Three German views* (pp. 68–78). Notre Dame, IN: University of Notre Dame Press.

Gaines, R. N. (1979). Identification and redemption in Lysias' "Against Eratosthenes." *Central States Speech Journal, 30,* 199–210.

Gaines, S. (1995). Relationships between members of cultural minorities. In J. T. Wood & S. Duck (Eds.), *Understanding relationship processes, 6: Off the beaten track understanding relationships.* Thousand Oaks, CA: Sage.

Galsworthy, T. (1994). Osteoporosis: Statistics, interviews, and prevention. In J. Sechzer, A. Griffin, & S. Pfallin (Eds.), *Forging a women's health research agenda: Policy issues for the 1990s* (pp. 158–163). New York: The New York Academy of Science.

Garfinkel, H. (1956). Some sociological concepts and methods for psychiatrists. *Psychiatric Research Reports, 6,* 181–195.

Garfinkel, H. (1967). *Studies in ethnomethodology.* Englewood Cliffs, NJ: Prentice-Hall.

Gergen, K. (1991). *The saturated self: Dilemmas of identity in contemporary life.* New York: Basic Books.

Gibson, C. (1970). Eugene Talmadge's use of identification during the 1934 gubernatorial campaign in Georgia. *Southern Speech Communication Journal, 35,* 342–349.

Glenn, L. D. (1990). *Health care communication between American Indian women and a White male doctor: A study of interaction at a public health care facility.* Unpublished doctoral dissertation, University of Oklahoma, Norman.

Glenn, P. J. (1989). Initiating shared laughter in multi-party conversation. *Western Journal of Speech Communication, 53*(2), 127–149.

Goffman, E. (1955). On face-work. *Psychiatry, 18,* 213–231.

Goffman, E. (1959). *Presentation of self in everyday life.* New York: Doubleday.

Goffman, E. (1967). *Interaction ritual.* New York: Pantheon Books.

Goffman, E. (1972). *Relations in public: Microstudies of the public order.* New York: Harper Collins.

Goffman, E. (1974). *Frame analysis: An essay on the organization of experience.* New York: Harper & Row.

Goldberg, R., Guadagnoli, E., Silliman, R., & Glicksman, A. (1990). Cancer patients' concerns: Congruence between patients and primary care physicians. *Journal of Cancer Education, 5*(3), 193–199.

Gorenberg, H., & White, A. (1991–1992). Off the pedestal and into the arena: Toward including women in experimental protocols. *Review of Law and Social Change, 20,* 205–246.

Greene, J. O., & Lindsey, A. E. (1989). Encoding processes in the production of multiple-goal messages. *Human Communication Research, 16,* 120–140.

Grimshaw, A. D. (1971). Sociolinguistics. In J. A. Fishman (Ed.), *Advances in the sociology of languages.* The Hague: Mouton.

Gumperz, J. (1971). *Language in social groups: Essays by John J. Gumperz.* Stanford: Stanford University Press.

Haas, J. S., Udvarheli, S., Epstein, A. M. (1993). The effect of health coverage for uninsured pregnant women and the use of cesarean section. *Journal of the American Medical Association, 270,* 61–64.

Hack, T. F., Degner, L. F., & Dyck, D. G. (1994). Relationship between preferences for decisional control and illness information among women with breast cancer: A quantitative and qualitative analysis. *Social Science Medicine, 39*(2), 279–289.

Haggard, A. (1989). *Handbook of patient education.* Rockville, MD: Aspen.

Halberstadt, A., & Saitta, M. (1987). Gender, nonverbal behavior, and perceived dominance: A test of the theory. *Journal of Personality and Social Psychology, 53,* 257–272.

Halvorson, G. (1993). *Strong medicine.* New York: Random House.

Haraway, D. (1988). Situated knowledge: The science question in feminism and the privilege of partial perspective. *Signs, 14,* 575–599.

Harding, S. (1991). *Whose science? Whose knowledge?: Thinking from women's lives.* Ithaca, NY: Cornell University Press.

Healy, B. (1991). The Yentl syndrome. *New England Journal of Medicine, 325,* 274–275.

Heath, C. (1986). *Body movement and speech in medical interaction.* Cambridge: Cambridge University Press.

Helms, D. T., Anderson, W. T., Meehan, A. J., & Rawls, A. W. (Eds.). (1989). *The interaction order: New directions in the study of social order.* New York: Irvington.

Hensbest, R. J., & Stewart, M. (1990). Patient centredness in the consultation. 2: Does it really make a difference? *Family Practice, 7*(1), 28–33.

Heritage, J. (1984). *Garfinkel and ethnomethodology.* Cambridge, MA: Polity.

Hilbert, R. A. (1990). Ethnomethodology and the micro–macro order. *American Sociological Review, 55,* 794–808.

Hilts, P. J. (1995, January 13). U.S. breast cancer deaths fell nearly 5 percent in three years. *The New York Times,* p. A17.

Holmes, H. B., & Purdy, L. M. (Eds.). (1992). *Feminist perspectives in medical ethics.* Bloomington: Indiana University Press.

How medicine mistreats women. (1994, October 26). *The Oprah Winfrey Show.* Chicago: Harpo Productions.

Hulka, B. S., Cassel, L. C., Kupper, L. L., & Burdette, J. A. (1976). Communication compliance, and concordance between physicians and patients with prescribed medications. *American Journal of Public Health, 66,* 847–853.

Humphrey, G. B., Littlewood, J. L., & Kamps, W. A. (1992). Physician/patient communication: A model considering the interaction of physicians' therapeutic strategy and patients' coping styles. *Journal of Cancer Education, 7*(2), 147–152.

Hunt, L. M., Jordan, B., Irwin, S., & Browner, C. H. (1989). Compliance and the patient's perspective: Controlling symptoms in everyday life. *Culture, Medicine, and Psychiatry, 13,* 315–334.

Huston, M., & Schwartz, P. (1995). Gendered dynamics in the romantic relationships of lesbians and gay men. In J. T. Wood (Ed.), *Gendered relationships* (pp. 163–176). Mountain View, CA: Mayfield.

Hymes, D. (1972). Models of the interaction of language and social life. In J. J. Gumperz & D. Hymes (Eds.), *Directions in sociolinguistics: The ethnography of communication* (pp. 38–71). New York: Holt, Rinehart & Winston.

Ivins, J. P., & Kent, G. G. (1993). Women's preferences for male or female gynecologists. *Journal of Reproductive and Infant Psychology, 11,* 209–214.

Jefferson, G. (1979). A technique for inviting laughter and its subsequent acceptance declination. In G. Psathas (Ed.), *Everyday language: Studies in ethnomethodology* (pp. 79–96). New York: Irvington.

Jefferson, G. (1984). On the organization of laughter in talk about troubles. In J. Heritage & J. Heritage (Eds.), *Structures of social action: Studies in conversation analysis* (pp. 346–369). Cambridge: Cambridge University Press.

Jones, C. M. (1994). *Supportive communication in physician-patient interviews: The case of the missing assessments.* Paper presented at the annual meeting of the Speech Communication Association, New Orleans, LA.

Jones, C. M. (in press). "That's a good sign": Encouraging assessments as a form of social support in medical-related encounters. *Health Communication.*

Joos, S. K., Hickam, D. H., & Borders, L. M. (1993). Patients' desires and satisfaction in general medicine clinics. *Public Health Reports, 108*(6), 751–759.

Kallen, D. J., & Stephenson, J. J. (1981). Perceived physician humaneness, patient attitude and satisfaction with the pill as a contraceptive. *Journal of Health and Social Behavior, 22,* 256–267.

Katovich, M. A. (1986). Temporal stages of situated activity and identity activation. In C. J. Couch, S. L. Saxton, & M. A. Katovich (Eds.), *Studies in symbolic interaction: A research annual: The Iowa School, Supplement 2 (Part B)* (pp. 329–352). Greenwich, CT: JAI.

Katz, J. (1984). *The silent world of doctor and patient.* London: The Free Press.

Kendall, J. (Ed.). (1990). *Combining service and learning.* Raleigh, NC: Publications Unlimited.

Keyser, H. H. (1984). *Women under the knife.* Philadelphia: George F. Stickley.

Khan, S. S., Nessim, S., Gray, R., Czer, L. S. Chaux, A., & Matloff, J. (1990). Increased mortality of women in coronary artery bypass surgery: Evidence for referral bias. *Annals of Internal Medicine, 112,* 561–567.

Kjernik, D., & Martinson, I. (Eds.). (1986). *Women in health: Life experiences and crises.* Philadelphia: Saunders.

Kjerulff, K., Langenberg, P., & Guzinski, G. (1993). The socioeconomic correlates of hysterectomies in the United States. *American Journal of Public Health, 83*(1), 106–108.

Klingle, R. S., & Burgoon, M. (1995). Patient compliance and satisfaction with physician influence attempts: A reinforcement expectancy approach to compliance-gaining over time. *Communication Research, 22*(2), 148–187.

Knorr-Cetina, K. D. (1981). Introduction: The micro-sociological challenge of macro-sociology: Towards a reconstruction of social theory and methodology. In K. D. Knorr-Cetina & A. V. Cicourel (Eds.), *Advances in social theory and methodology: Towards an integration of micro- and macro-sociologies* (pp. 1–47). Boston: Routledge & Kegan Paul.

Kolata, G. (1993, May 5). Why do so many women have breasts removed needlessly? *The New York Times,* p. C13.

Kolb, D. (1984). *Experiential learning.* Englewood, NJ: Prentice-Hall.

Korsch, B. M., Gozzi, E. K., & Negrete, V. F. (1968). Gaps in doctor–patient interaction and patient satisfaction. *Pediatrics, 42,* 855–870.

Korsch, B. M., & Negrete, V. F. (1972). Doctor–patient communication. *Scientific America, 227,* 66–74.

Kraft, R., & Swadener, M. (Eds.). (1994). *Building community: Service learning in the academic disciplines.* Denver: Colorado Campus Compact.

Kramarae, C. (1996). Classified information: Race, class, and (always) gender. In J. T. Wood (Ed.), *Gendered relationships* (pp. 20–38). Mountain View, CA: Mayfield.

Kreps, G. L. (1993). Relational communication in health care. *Southern Speech Communication Journal, 53,* 344–359.

Kreps, G. L., & Query, J., Jr. (1990). Health communication and interpersonal competence. In G. M. Phillilps & J. T. Wood (Eds.), *Speech communication: Essays to commemorate the 75th anniversary of the Speech Communication Association* (pp. 293–323). Carbondale: Southern Illinois Press.

Krulewitch, H. (1980). Changing the doctor–patient relationship: A doctor's point of view. *Holistic Health Review, 3*(4), 284–288.

Kurata, J. H., Nogawa, A. N., Phillips, D. M., Hoffman, S., & Werblun, M. N. (1992). Patient and provider satisfaction with medical care. *The Journal of Family Practice, 35*(2), 176–179.

Lakoff, R. (1975). *Language and women's place.* New York: Harper & Row.

Lamas, G. A., Pashos, C. L., Normand, S. T., & McNeil, B. (1995). Permanent pacemaker selection and subsequent survival in elderly Medicare patients. *Circulation, 91,* 1063–1069.

Landen, M., & Lampert, K. (1992). Cervical cancer screening: At the patient's or the health system's convenience? *The IHS Primary Care Provider, 10,* 174–179.

LaRosa, J. (1994). Office of research on women's health: National Institutes of Health and the women's health agenda. In J. Sechzer, A. Griffin, & S. Pfallin (Eds.), *Forging a women's health research agenda: Policy issues for the 1990's* (pp. 196–204). New York: The New York Academy of Science.

Laurence, L., & Weinhouse, B. (1994). *Outrageous practices: The alarming truth about how medicine mistreats women.* New York: Fawcett Columbine.

Leff, M. C. (1973). Redemptive identification: Cicero's catilinarian orations. In G. P. Mohrmann, C. J. Stewart, & D. Ochs (Eds.), *Explorations in rhetorical criticism* (pp. 158–177). University Park: The Pennsylvania State University.

Legato, M. (1994). Cardiovascular disease in women: What's different? What's new? What's unresolved? In J. Sechzer, A. Griffin, & S. Pfallin (Eds.), *Forging a women's health research agenda: Policy issues for the 1990's* (pp. 147–157). New York: The New York Academy of Science.

Leserman, L., & Luke, S. (1982). An evaluation of an innovative approach to teaching the pelvic examination to medical students. *Women and Health, 6,* 37–55.

Levinson, R. M., McCollum, K. T., & Kutner, N. G. (1984). Gender homophily in preferences for physicians. *Sex Roles, 10,* 315–325.

Lewin, E., & Oleson, V. (Eds.). (1985). *Women, health, and healing: Toward a new perspective.* New York: Tavistock.

Lim, T. (1994). Facework and interpersonal relationships. In S. Ting-Toomey (Ed.), *The challenge of facework* (pp. 209–230). Albany: The State University of New York Press.

Lipsitt, D. (1982). The painful woman: Complaints symptoms and illness. In M. T. Notman & C. Nadelson (Eds.), *The Woman Patient* (pp. 147–171). New York: Plenum.

Livingston, R., & Ostrow, D. (1978). Professional patient-instructors in the teaching of the pelvic examination. *American Journal of Obstetrics and Gynecology, 132,* 64–67.

Low, K. G., Joliceour, M. R., Colman, R. A., Stone, L. E., & Fleisher, C. L. (1994). Women participants in research: Assessing progress. *Women and Health, 22,* 79–98.

Lurie, N., Slater, J., McGovern, P., Ekstrum, J., Quam, L., & Margolis, K. (1993). Preventive care for women: Does the sex of the physician matter? *New England Journal of Medicine, 329,* 478–482.

Majeroni, B. A., Karuza, J., Wade, C., McCreadie, M., & Calkins, E. (1993). Gender of physicians and patients and preventive care for community-based older adults. *Journal of the American Board of Family Practice, 6,* 359–365.

Mandelbaum, J. (1987). Interpersonal activities in conversational storytelling. *Western Journal of Speech Communication, 53,* 114–126.

Mandelbaum, J. (1990). Communication phenomena as solutions to interactional problems. In J. Anderson (Ed.), *Communication yearbook 13* (pp. 255–267). Newbury Park, CA: Sage.

Mandelbaum, J., & Pomerantz, A. (1991). What drives social action? In K. Tracy (Ed.), *Understanding face-to-face interaction: Issues linking goals and discourse* (pp. 151–166). Hillsdale, NJ: Lawrence Erlbaum Associates.

Manning, P. (1970). Talking and becoming: A view of organizational socialization. In J. D. Douglas (Ed.), *Understanding everyday life: Toward the reconstruction of sociological knowledge* (pp. 239–256). Chicago: Aldine.

Mark, D. B., Shaw, L. K., DeLong, E. R., Califf, R. M., & Pryor, D. B. (1994). Absence of sex bias in referral of patients for cardiac catheterization. *New England Journal of Medicine, 330,* 1101–1106.

Markova, I., & Foppa, K. (Eds.). (1991). *Asymmetries in dialogue.* Savage, MD: Barnes & Noble Books.

Maseide, P. (1981). Sincerity may frighten the patient: Medical dilemmas in patient care. *Journal of Pragmatics, 5,* 145–167.

Mastroianni, A. C., Faden, R., & Federman, D. (Eds.). (1994a). *Women and health research: Ethics and legal issues of including women in clinical studies* (Vol. 1). Washington, DC: National Academy Press.

Mastroianni, A. C., Faden, R., & Federman, D. (Eds.). (1994b). *Women and health research: Ethics and legal issues of including women in clinical studies* (Vol. 2). Washington, DC: National Academy Press.

Maynard, C., Litwin, P. E., Martin, J. S., & Weaver, W. D. (1992). Gender differences in the treatment and outcome of acute myocardial infarction. *Archives of Internal Medicine, 152,* 972–976.

McHugh, P. (1968). *Defining the situation: The organization of meaning in social interaction.* Indianapolis, IN: Bobbs-Merrill.

McIntosh, J. (1976). *Communication and awareness in a cancer ward.* London: Croom Helm.

McNeilis, K. S., & Thompson, T. L. (1995). The impact of relational control on patient compliance in dentist/patient interactions. In G. Kreps & D. O'Hair (Eds.), *Communication and health outcomes* (pp. 57–72). Cresskill, NJ: Hampton Press.

McNeilis, K., Thompson, T., & O'Hair, D. (1995). Implications of relational communication for therapeutic discourse. In G. Morris & R. Chenail (Eds.), *The talk of the clinic* (pp. 291–314). Hillsdale, NJ: Lawrence Erlbaum Associates.

Meewesen, L., Schaap, C., & Van Der Staak, C. (1991) Verbal analysis of doctor-patient communication. *Social Science Medicine, 32*(10), 1143–1150.

Menken, M. (1992). What improved my patient communications? Getting sued. *Medical Economics, 69*(7), 54–56.

Miles, A. (1991). *Women, health, and medicine.* Philadelphia: Open University Press.

Millar, F. E., & Rogers, L. E. (1976). A relational approach to interpersonal communication. In G. R. Miller (Ed.), *Explorations in interpersonal communication* (pp. 87–103). Beverly Hills, CA: Sage.

Millar, F. E., Rogers, L. E., & Bavelas, J. (1984). Identifying patterns of verbal conflict in interpersonal dynamics. *Western Journal of Communication, 48,* 231–246.

Mishler, E. G. (1984). *The discourse of medicine: Dialectics of medical interviews.* Norwood, NJ: Ablex.

Modaff, D. P. (1995). *Enacting asymmetry in the opening moments of the doctor-patient interview.* Unpublished doctoral dissertation, University of Texas, Austin.

Montgomery, B. (1993). *Healing through communication.* Newbury Park, CA: Sage.

Morris, G. H., White, C. H., & Itis, R. (1994). Well, ordinarily I would, but: Reexamining the nature of accounts for problematic events. *Research on Language and Social Interaction, 27*(2), 123–144.

Muller, C. F. (1992). *Health care and gender.* New York: Russell Sage.

National Center for Health Statistics. (1991). *National hospital discharge data, 1979–1984.* Hyattsville, MD: U.S. Department of Health and Human Services.

National Institutes of Health. (1996a). *Consensus Development Conference Statement on Cervical Cancer.* Bethesda, MD: Author.

National Institutes of Health. (1996b, April 6). *NIH panel urges wider screening for cervical cancer* (news release). Bethesda, MD: Author.

NBC News Transcripts. (1995, January 17). Discussion of new awareness of women's risk of heart attacks. *Dateline NBC.*

Nechas, E., & Foley, D. (1994). *Unequal treatment: What you don't know about how women are mistreated by the medical community.* New York: Simon & Schuster.

O'Hair, D. (1989). Dimensions of relational communication and control during physician-patient interactions. *Health Communication, 1*(2), 97–115.

O'Hair, D., O'Hair, M., Southward, G. M., & Krayer, K. J. (1987). Physician communication and patient compliance. *The Journal of Compliance in Health, 2*(2), 125–129.

Parks, M. R. (1977). Relational communication: Theory and research. *Human Communication Research, 3*(4), 372–381.

Parsons, T. (1951). *The social system.* New York: The Free Press.

Payne, D. (1995). Kenneth Burke and contemporary criticism. *Text and Performance Quarterly, 15,* 333–347.

Penman, R. (1994). Facework in communication: Conceptual and moral challenges. In S. Ting-Toomey (Ed.), *The challenge of facework* (pp. 15–46). Albany: State University of New York Press.

Petticrew, M., McKee, M., & Jones, J. (1993). Coronary artery surgery: Are women discriminated against? *British Medical Journal, 306,* 1164–1166.

Pfallin, S. C. (1994). Future directions for women's health. In J. Sechzer, A. Griffin, & S. Pfallin (Eds.), *Forging a women's health research agenda: Policy issues for the 1990's. Annals of the New York Academy of Sciences, 736.* New York: The New York Academy of Science.

Phillips, G. M., & Jones, J. A. (1991). Medical compliance: Patient or physician responsibility? *American Behavioral Scientist, 34*(6), 756–767.

Pilote, L. (1994). Presentation to the American College of Cardiology, Atlanta, GA.

Pollner, M. (1987). *Mundane reason.* Cambridge: Cambridge University Press.

Pomerantz, A. (1989). Epilogue. *Western Journal of Speech Communication, 53,* 242–246.

Pomerantz, A. (1990). Chautauqua: On the validity and generalizability of conversational analysis methods. *Communication Monographs, 57,* 231–235.

Ragan, S. L. (1990). Verbal play and multiple goals in the gynecologic exam interaction. *Journal of Language and Social Psychology, 9,* 67–84.

Ragan, S. L., Beck, C., & White, M. D. (1995). Educating the patient: Interactive learning in an OB-GYN context. In G. H. Morris & R. J. Chenail (Eds.), *The talk of the clinic: Explorations in the analysis of medical and therapeutic discourse* (pp. 185–208). Hillsdale, NJ: Lawrence Erlbaum Associates.

Ragan, S. L., & Glenn, L. D. (1990). Communication and gynecologic health care. In D. O'Hair & G. Kreps (Eds.), *Applied communication theory and research* (pp. 313–330). Hillsdale, NJ: Lawrence Erlbaum Associates.

Ragan, S. L., & Pagano, M. (1987). Communicating with female patients: Affective interaction during contraceptive counseling and gynecologic exam. *Women's Studies in Communication, 10,* 45–57.

Rinzler, C. A. (1993). *Estrogen and breast cancer: A warning to women.* New York: Macmillan.

Roberts, H. (1981). Women and their doctors: Power and powerlessness in the research process. In H. Roberts (Ed.), *Doing feminist research* (pp. 7–29). Boston: Routledge & Kegan Paul.

Rogers, L. E. (1981). Symmetry and complementarity: Evolution and evaluation of an idea. In C. Wilder-Mott & J. H. Weakland (Eds.), *Rigor and imagination: Essays from the legacy of Gregory Bateson* (pp. 231–251). New York: Praeger.

Rogers, L. E. (1989). Relational communication processes and patterns. In B. Dervin, L. Grossberg, B. O'Keefe, & E. Wartella (Eds.), *Rethinking communication: Vol. 2. Paradigm exemplars* (pp. 280–290). Newbury Park, CA: Sage.

Rogers, L. E., & Bagarozzi, D. A. (1983). An overview of relational communication and implications for therapy. In D. Bagarozzi, A. Jurich, & R. Jackson (Eds.), *Marital and family therapy: New perspectives in theory, research and practice* (pp. 48–78). New York: Human Sciences Press.

Rogers, L., & Farace, R. V. (1995). Analysis of relational communication in dyads: New measurement procedures. *Human Communication Research, 1*(3), 222–239.

Rogers, L. E., & Millar, F. E. (1988). Relational communication. In S. Duck (Ed.), *Handbook of personal relationships* (pp. 289–305). New York: Wiley.

Roter, D. (1979). Altering patient participation in the patient-provider interaction: The effects of patient question-asking on the quality of interaction, satisfaction, and compliance. *Health Education Monographs, 5,* 281–330.

Roter, D. L. (1983). Physician/patient communication: Transmission of information and patient effects. *Michigan State Medical Journal, 32*(4), 260–265.

Roter, D. L. (1984). Patient question asking in physician-patient interaction. *Health Psychology, 3*(5), 395–409.

Roter, D. L., Lipkin, M., Jr., & Korsgaard, A. (1991). Sex differences in patients' and physicians' communication during primary care medical visits. *Medical Care, 29*(11), 1083–1093.

Rowland-Morin, P. A., & Carroll, J. G. (1990). Verbal communication skills and patient satisfaction: A study of doctor-patient interviews. *Evaluation and the Health Professions, 13*(2), 169–185.

Sacks, H. (1974). An analysis of the course of a joke's telling in conversation. In R. Bauman & J. Sherzer (Eds.), *Explorations in the ethnography of speaking* (pp. 337–353). Cambridge: University of Cambridge Press.

Sacks, H. (1984). Notes on methodology. In J. M. Atkinson & J. C. Heritage (Eds.), *Structures of social actions* (pp. 21–27). Cambridge: Cambridge University Press.

Sacks, H. (1992a). *Lectures on conversation* (Vol. 1). Oxford, England: Blackwell.

Sacks, H. (1992b). *Lectures on conversation* (Vol. 2). Oxford, England: Blackwell.

Sacks, H., Schegloff, E., & Jefferson, G. (1974). A simplest systematics for the organization of turn-taking for conversation. *Language, 50,* 696–735.

Sanbonmatsu, A. (1971). Darrow and Rorke's use of Burkeian identification strategies in New York vs. Gitlow (1920). *Speech Monographs, 38,* 36–48.

Sanders, R. E. (1991). The two-way relationship between talk in social interactions and actors' goals and plans. In K. Tracy (Ed.), *Understanding face-to-face interaction: Issues linking goals and discourse* (pp. 167–188). Hillsdale, NJ: Lawrence Erlbaum Associates.

Satterlund-Larsson, U., Johanson, M., & Svardsudd, K. (1994). Sensitive patient-doctor communications relating to the breast and prostate. *Sensitive Patient Communication, 9*(1), 19–25.

Schain, W. S. (1990). Physician–patient communication about breast cancer: A challenge for the 1990s. *Surgical Clinics of North America, 70*(4), 917–936.

Schegloff, E. A. (1980). Preliminaries to preliminaries: "Can I ask you a question?" *Sociological Inquiry, 50,* 104–152.

Schegloff, E. A. (1982). Discourse as an interactional achievement: Some uses of "uh huh" and other things that come between sentences. In D. Tannen (Ed.), *Analyzing discourse: Text and talk* (pp. 71–93). Washington, DC: Georgetown University Press.

Schegloff, E. A. (1986). The routine as achievement. *Human Studies, 9,* 111–151.

Schegloff, E. A. (1987). Analyzing single episodes of interaction: An exercise in conversation analysis. *Social Psychology Quarterly, 50,* 101–114.

Schegloff, E. A., Jefferson, G., & Sacks, H. (1977). The preference for self-correction in the organisation of repair in conversation. *Language, 53,* 361–382.

Schegloff, E. A., & Sacks, H. (1973). Opening up closings. *Semiotica, 7,* 289–327.

Schutz, A. (1962). *Collected papers: Vol. 1.* The Hague: Mouton.

Schutz, A. (1970). *On phenomenology and social relations.* Chicago: University of Chicago Press.

Sechzer, J., Griffin, A., & Pfallin, S. (Eds.). (1994). *Forging a women's health research agenda: Policy issues for the 1990's. Annals of the New York Academy of Sciences, 736.* New York: The New York Academy of Science.

Seidman, S. (Ed.). (1994). *The postmodern turn: New perspectives on social theory.* New York: Cambridge University Press.

Shapiro, M. C., Najman, J. M., Chang, A., Keeping, J. D., Morrison, J., & Western, J. S. (1983). Information control and the exercise of power in the obstetrical encounter. *Social Science and Medicine, 17,* 139–146.

Sharf, B. (1988). Teaching patients to speak up: Past and future trends. *Patient Education and Counseling, 11,* 95–108.

Shaw, L. J., Miller, D., Romeis, J. C., Kargl, D., Younis, L. T., & Chaitman, B. R. (1994). Gender differences in the non-invasive evaluation management with suspected coronary artery disease. *Annals of Internal Medicine, 120,* 559–566.

Sherwin, S. (1992). *No longer patient: Feminist ethics and health care.* Philadelphia: Temple University Press.

Shimanoff, S. (1988). Degree of emotional expressiveness as a function of face-needs, gender, and interpersonal relationship. *Communication Reports, 1,* 43–53.

Shimanoff, S. (1994). Gender perspectives on facework: Simplistic stereotypes vs. complex realities. In S. Ting-Toomey (Ed.), *The challenge of facework: Cross-cultural and interpersonal issues* (pp. 159–208). Albany: State University of New York Press.

Shotter, J., & Gergen, K. J. (1994). Social construction: Knowledge, self, others, and continuing the conversation. In S. Deetz (Ed.), *Communication yearbook 17* (pp. 3–33). Newbury Park, CA: Sage.

Silverman, D. (1987). *Communication and medical practice.* London: Sage.

Sluzki, C., & Beavin, J. (1965). Simetria y complementaridad: Una definicion operacional y una tipologia de parejas [Symmetry and complimentarity: An operational definition and a typology of dyads]. *Acta Psiquiatrica y Psychologica de America Latina, 11,* 321–330.

Smilkstein, G., DeWolfe, D., Erwin, M., McIntyre, M., & Shuford, D. (1980). A biomedical-psychosocial format for an educational pelvic examination. *Journal of Medical Education, 55,* 630–663.

Smith, D. H., & Pettegrew, L. S. (1986). Mutual persuasion as a model for doctor–patient communication. *Theoretical Medicine, 7,* 127–146.

Smith, J. M. (1992). *Women and doctors.* New York: Atlantic Monthly.

Smith-DuPre, A. A., & Beck, C. (1996). Enabling patients and physicians to pursue multiple goals in health care encounters: A case study. *Health Communication, 8,* 73–90.

Solomon, A. (1991, May 14). The politics of breast cancer. *Village Voice,* pp. 25–27.

Spelman, E. (1988). *Inessential women: Problems of exclusion in feminist thought.* Boston: Beacon Press.

Squyres, W. D. (Ed.). (1980). *Patient education: An inquiry into the state of the art* (Vol. 4). New York: Springer.

Squyres, W. D. (1985). *Patient education and health promotion in medical care.* Palo Alto: Mayfield.

Starr, C. (1992, April 6). Women and heart disease: A connection scorned? *Drug Topics,* pp. 35–44.

Steele, G. D., Winchester, D. P., Menck, H. R., & Murphy, G. D. (1993). Clinical highlights from the National Cancer database: 1993. *CA-A Cancer Journal for Clinicians, 43,* 71–82.

Steingart, R., & Wassertheil-Smoller, S. (1992). Coronary artery disease in women: Under diagnosed and under treated. *Journal of Myocardial Ischein, 4,* 13–22.

Stewart, M. A. (1984). What is a successful doctor–patient interview? A study of interactions and outcomes. *Social Science Medicine, 19*(2), 167–175.

Stone, G. C. (1979). Patient compliance and the role of the expert. *Journal of Social Issues, 35,* 34–59.

Street, R. L. (1989). Patient's satisfaction with dentists' communicative style. *Health Communication, 1*(3), 137–154.

Street, R. L., & Wiemann, J. M. (1987). Differences in how physicians and patients perceive physicians' relational communication. *The Southern Speech Journal, 53,* 420–440.

Summey, P., & Hurst, M. (1986). Ob/gyn on the rise: The evolution of professional ideology in the twentieth century—part 2. *Women and Health, 11*(2), 103–122.

Tannen, D. (1990). *You just don't understand: Women and men in conversation.* New York: William Morrow.

Tannen, D. (1994). *Gender and discourse.* New York: Oxford University Press.

Tardy, R. W. (1994). *Health information-seeking as a job requirement for motherhood: An ethnographic and network analysis of the business of stay-at-home moms.* Unpublished doctoral dissertation, Ohio University, Athens.

Taylor, C. (1994). Gender equity in research. *Journal of Women's Health, 3*(3), 143–153.

Ten Have, P. (1991). Talk and institution: A reconsideration of the "asymmetry" of doctor-patient interaction. In D. Boden & D. H. Zimmerman (Eds.), *Talk and social structure* (pp. 138–163). Berkeley: University of California Press.

Thomas, S., & Finck, A. C. (1994). Women's health: Early detection and screening practices for breast and cervical cancer. *Journal of the Louisiana State Medical Society, 146,* 152–158.

Thompson, T. L. (1984). The invisible helping hand: The role of communication in the health and social service professions. *Communication Quarterly, 32*(2), 148–163.

Thompson, T. L. (1990). Patient health care: Issues in interpersonal communication. In E. B. Ray & L. Donohew (Eds.), *Communication and health: Systems and applications* (pp. 27–50). Hillsdale, NJ: Lawrence Erlbaum Associates.

Thompson, T. L., & Gillotti, C. (1993). From labor to NICU: The journey of a premature baby and her parents. In E. B. Ray (Ed.), *Case studies in health communication* (pp. 87–100). Hillsdale, NJ: Lawrence Erlbaum Associates.

Ting-Toomey, S. (Ed.). (1994). *The challenge of facework: Cross-cultural and interpersonal issues.* Albany: State University of New York Press.

Ting-Toomey, S., & Cocroft, B. (1994). Face and facework: Theoretical and research issues. In S. Ting-Toomey (Ed.), *The challenge of facework* (pp. 307–340). Albany: State University of New York Press.

Todd, A. D. (1989). *Intimate adversaries: Cultural conflict between doctors and women patients.* Philadelphia: University of Pennsylvania Press.

Todd, A. D. (1993). Exploring women's experiences: Power and resistance in medical discourse. In A. D. Todd & S. Fisher (Eds.), *The social organization of doctor–patient communication* (pp. 267–285). Norwood, NJ: Ablex.

Todd, A. D., & Fisher, S. (Eds.). (1993). *The social organizaiton of doctor–patient communication.* Norwood, NJ: Ablex.

Townsend, J. (1992). *Strenthening research in academic OB/GYN departments.* Washington, DC: National Academy Press.

Tracy, K. (1984). The effect of multiple goals on conversational relevance and topic shift. *Communication Monographs, 51,* 274–287.

Tracy, K. (1990). The many faces of facework. In H. Giles & P. Robinson (Eds.), *Handbook of language and social psychology* (pp. 209–223). London: Wiley.

Tracy, K. (1991a). Introduction: Linking communicator goals with discourse. In K. Tracy (Ed.), *Understanding face-to-face interaction: Linking goals with discourse* (pp. 1–20). Hillsdale, NJ: Lawrence Erlbaum Associates.

Tracy, K. (Ed.). (1991b). *Understanding face-to-face interaction: Linking goals with discourse.* Hillsdale, NJ: Lawrence Erlbaum Associates.

Tracy, K., & Baratz, S. (1994). The case for case studies of facework. In S. Ting-Toomey (Ed.), *The challenge of facework* (pp. 287–306). Albany: The State University of New York Press.

Tracy, K., & Carjuzaa, J. (1993). Identity enactments in intellectual discussion. *Journal of Language and Social Psychology, 12*(3), 171–194.

Tracy, K., & Coupland, N. (1990). Multiple goals in discourse: An overview of issues. *Journal of Language and Social Psychology, 9,* 1–12.

Tracy, K., & Naughton, J. (1994). The identity work of questioning in intellectual discussion. *Communication Monographs, 61,* 281–302.

Treichler, P., Frankel, R. M., & Kramarae, C. (1984). Problems and problems: Power relationships in a medical encounter. In C. Kramarae, M. Schultz, & W. O'Barr (Eds.), *Language and power* (pp. 62–89). Beverly Hills, CA: Sage.

Trenholm, S. (1991). *Human communication theory* (2nd ed.). Englewood Cliffs, NJ: Prentice-Hall.

Turner, J. H. (1985). The concept of "action" in sociological analysis. In G. Seebass & R. Tuomela (Eds.), *Social action* (pp. 61–87). Dordrecht, The Netherlands: Reidel.

U.S. Bureau of the Census. (1994). *Statistical abstract of the United States: 1994* (14th ed.). Washington, DC: U.S. Department of Commerce, Economics and Statistics Administration.

von Friederichs-Fitzwater, M. M., Callahan, E. J., Flynn, N., & Williams, J. (1991). Relational control in physician–patient encounters. *Health Communication, 3*(1), 17–36.

Waitzkin, H. (1984). Doctor–patient communication: Clinical implications of social scientific research. *Journal of the American Medical Association, 252*(17), 2441–2446.

Waitzkin, H. (1985). Information giving in medical care. *Journal of Health and Social Behavior, 26,* 81–101.

Waller, K. (1988). Women doctors for women patients? *British Journal of Medical Psychology,*
61, 125–135.

Watzlawick, P., Bavelas, J., & Jackson, D. (1967). *Pragmatics of human communication.* New
York: Norton.

Weaver, J. L., & Garrett, S. D. (1982). Sexism and racism in the American health care industry.
In E. Fee (Ed.), *Women and health: The politics of sex in medicine* (pp. 79–104). Farmingdale, NY: Baywood.

Weijts, W. (1994). Responsible health communication: Taking control of our lives. *American*
Behavioral Scientist, 38(2), 257–270.

Weijts, W., Widdershoven, G., & Kok, G. (1991). Anxiety-scenarios in communication during
gynecological consultations. *Patient Education and Counseling, 18,* 149–163.

Weijts, W., Widdershoven, G., Kok, G., & Tomlow, P. (1993). Patients' information-seeking
actions and physicians' responses in gynecological consultations. *Qualitative Health Research, 3*(4), 398–429.

Weisensee, M. (1986). Women's health perceptions in a male-dominated medical world. In D.
Kjernik & I. Martinson (Eds.), *Women in health and illness: Life experiences and crises* (pp.
19–33). Philidelphia: Saunders.

Weisman, C. S. (1986, July/August). Women and their health care providers: A matter of communication. *Public Health Reports Supplement,* 147–151.

Weisman, C. S., & Teitelbaum, M. A. (1985). Physician gender and the physician–patient relationship: Recent evidence and revelant questions. *Social Science Medicine, 20*(11), 1119–
1127.

Weiss, L., & Meadow, R. (1979). Women's attitudes towards gynecological practices. *Obstetrics*
and Gynecology, 54, 110–114.

West, C. (1984). When the doctor is a "lady": Power, status and gender in physician–patient
encounters. *Symbolic Interaction, 7*(1), 87–106.

West, C. (1993a). "Ask me no questions . . .": An analysis of queries and replies in physician-
patient dialogues. In S. Fisher & A. D. Todd (Eds.), *The social organization of doctor-patient
communication* (pp. 127–160). Norwood, NJ: Ablex.

West, C. (1993b). Reconceptualizing gender in physician-patient relationships. *Social Science*
Medicine, 36(1), 57–66.

West, C., & Zimmerman, D. (1983). Small insults: A study of interruptions in cross-sex conversations with unacquainted persons. In B. Thorne, C. Kramarae, & H. Henley (Eds.), *Language,*
gender, and society (pp. 102–217). Rowley, MA: Newbury House.

West, S. (1994). *The hysterectomy hoax.* New York: Doubleday.

What every woman should know. (1993, May 12). *The Oprah Winfrey Show.* Chicago: Harpo
Productions.

Wheeless, V. E. (1987). Female patient and physician communication and discussion of gynecological health care issues. *The Southern Speech Communication Journal, 52,* 198–211.

White, P. (1993). Women and smoking. In A. McPherson (Ed.), *Women's problems in general*
practice (pp. 469–483). Oxford, England: Oxford University Press.

Wieder, D. L., & Pratt, S. (1990). On being a recognizable Indian among Indians. In D. Carbaugh
(Ed.), *Cultural communication and intercultural contact* (pp. 45–64). Hillsdale, NJ:
Lawrence Erlbaum Associates.

Wiener, C., Fagerhaugh, S., Strauss, A., & Suczek, B. (1980, September/October). Patient power
complex issues need complex answers. *Social Policy,* 30–38.

Wilder, C. (1979). The Palo Alto group: Difficulties and directions of the interactional view for
human communication research. *Human Communication Research, 5,* 171–186.

Wilder, C., & Collins, S. (1994). Patterns of interaction paradoxes. In W. R. Cupach & B. H.
Spitzberg (Eds.), *The dark side of interpersonal communication* (pp. 83–104). Hillsdale, NJ:
Lawrence Erlbaum Associates.

Wilder-Mott, C. (1981). Rigor and imagination. In C. Wilder-Mott & J. H. Weakland (Eds.), *Rigor and imagination: Essays from the legacy of Gregory Bateson* (pp. 5–42). New York: Praeger.

Wilder-Mott, C., & Weakland, J. H. (Eds.) (1981). *Rigor and imagination: Essays from the legacy of Gregory Bateson*. New York: Praeger.

Wilkins, C. A. (1996). *An ethnographic study of the emergence of culture in two merging health care organizations*. Unpublished doctoral dissertation, Ohio University, Athens.

Wilson, T. (1970). Normative and interpretive paradigms in sociology. In J. D. Douglas (Ed.), *Understanding everyday life: Toward the reconstruction of sociological knowledge* (pp. 221–238). Chicago: Aldine.

Winefield, H. R., & Murrell, T. G. C. (1991). Speech patterns and satisfaction in diagnostic and prescriptive stages of general practice consultations. *British Journal of Medical Psychology, 64*, 103–115.

Wolinsky, F. D. (1980). *The sociology of health, principles, professions and issues*. Boston: Little Brown.

Wood, J. T. (1996). *Gender relationships*. Mountain View, CA: Mayfield.

Young, M., & Klingle, R. (1996). Silent partners in medical care: A cross-cultural study of patient participation. *Health Communication, 8*(1), 29–54.

Zimmerman, D. H., & West, C. (1975). Sex roles, interruptions and silences in conversation. In B. Thorne & N. Henley (Eds.), *Language and sex: Difference and dominance* (pp. 105–129). Rowley, MA: Newbury House.

Zimmerman, D., & Pollner, M. (1970). The everyday world as phenomenon. In J. Douglas (Ed.), *Understanding everyday life: Toward the reconstruction of sociological knowledge* (pp. 80–103). Chicago: Aldine.

Zimmerman, R. S. (1988). The dental appointment and patient behavior. *Medical Care, 26*, 403–414.

Author Index

Subject Index

Printed and bound by CPI Group (UK) Ltd, Croydon, CR0 4YY

17/10/2024

01775656-0003